FIFTH EDITION

ADVANCED FETAL MONITORING COURSE

Student Materials

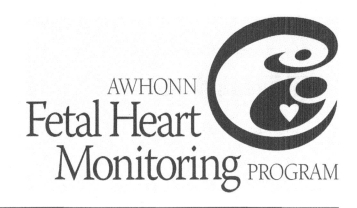

AWHONN
Fetal Heart
Monitoring PROGRAM

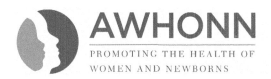

AWHONN
PROMOTING THE HEALTH OF
WOMEN AND NEWBORNS

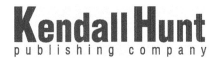

Kendall Hunt
publishing company

Cover image © Shutterstock, Inc.

Kendall Hunt
publishing company

www.kendallhunt.com
Send all inquiries to:
4050 Westmark Drive
Dubuque, IA 52004-1840

Copyright © 1999, 2001, 2006, 2010, and 2017 by Association of Women's Health, Obstetric and Neonatal Nurses

ISBN 978-1-5249-3309-8

Published in the United States of America

CONTENTS

Target Audience

The Advanced Fetal Heart Monitoring Course is based on an educational design that incorporates critical thinking and decision making and is specifically designed for clinicians with previous fetal heart monitoring (FHM) experience. Residents and physicians may also participate in the course. Although prior completion of the Intermediate Fetal Heart Monitoring Course is not a requirement for participation in the AWHONN Advanced Fetal Heart Monitoring Course, AWHONN strongly recommends completion of fetal monitoring education and intrapartum clinical experience prior to attendance. To facilitate successful completion of the course, participants are expected, prior to attending the course, to review the current edition of the book *Fetal Heart Monitoring Principles and Practices text prior to attending the course*. Although the content of this course is comprehensive, specific patient care responsibilities vary according to institution, state, province or region. Participants in this course are advised to be familiar with their organizational/institutional responsibilities, as well as competence criteria and measurement.

Acknowledgment of Commercial Support

This CNE/CME activity has been created without commercial support.

Sponsorship and Co-Providership Statements

The CNE activity is provided by the Association of Women's Health, Obstetric and Neonatal Nurses (AWHONN) in collaboration with co-provider, Professional Education Services Group (PESG).

This activity has been planned and implemented in accordance with the essential areas and policies of the Accreditation Council for Continuing Medical Education (ACCME) through the joint sponsorship of the Professional Education Services Group (PESG) and the Association of Women's Health, Obstetric and Neonatal Nurses (AWHONN). The Professional Education Services Group is accredited by the ACCME to provide continuing medical education for physicians.

Learning Objectives

At the conclusion of this continuing education activity, participants will:

- Describe physiologic principles of maternal and fetal oxygen transfer as they apply to principles of fetal heart monitoring.
- Recognize fetal cardiac arrhythmia patterns and describe potential outcomes associated with these patterns.
- Analyze complex case studies and tracings utilizing standardized terminology.
- Apply perinatal risk management principles, communication techniques and documentation strategies related to complex and challenging patient care scenarios.

Content Validation Statement

It is the policy of AWHONN and PESG to review and certify that the content contained in this CNE/CME activity is based on sound, scientific, evidence-based clinical practice. All recommendations in this CNE/CME activity are based on evidence that is accepted within the profession of medicine as adequate justification for their indications and contraindications in the care of patients. AWHONN and PESG further assert that all scientific research referred to, reported or used in this CNE/CME activity in support of or justification of a patient care recommendation conforms to the generally accepted standards of experimental design, data collection and analysis. Moreover, AWHONN and PESG establish that the content contained herein conforms to the definition of CNE as presented by the American Nurses Credentialing Center (ANCC) and the definition of CME as presented by the Accreditation Council for Continuing Medical Education (ACCME).

Disclosure Statement

It is the policy of AWHONN and PESG that the faculty and program planners and developers disclose real or apparent conflicts of interest relating to the topics of this education activity. Detailed disclosures, if applicable, will be made available during the live course.

Conflict of Interest Resolution Statement

When individuals in a position to control content have reported financial, professional or personal relationships with one or more commercial interests, AWHONN and PESG will resolve such conflicts to ensure that the presentation is free from commercial bias. The content of this presentation was vetted by the following mechanisms and modified as required to meet this standard:

- Content peer review by external topic expert
- Content validation by external topic expert and internal AWHONN and PESG clinical staff

  Educational Peer Review Disclosure PESG reports the following:

- **George J. Vuturo, RPh, PhD**
  Vice President of Medical Affairs/CME Director
  Dr. Vuturo has no relevant financial relationships to disclose.
- **Karen Langston, MSN, RNC-OB, C-EFM**
  has no relevant financial relationships to disclose.
- **Cindy Cochrane MS, RNC-OB, WHNP-BC**
  has no relevant financial relationships to disclose.
- **Christina L Rust, DNP, MSN, RNC-OB, C-EFM**
  has no relevant financial relationships to disclose.
- **Dr. John W. Caravello**
  has no relevant financial relationships to disclose.
- **Carol Elaine Brown, RN, BC, MN, E-EFM**
  Nurse Program Development Specialist, AWHONN
  Ms. Brown has no relevant financial relationships to disclose.

Accreditation Information

Association of Women's Health, Obstetric and Neonatal Nurses is accredited as a provider of continuing nursing education by the American Nurses Credentialing Center's Commission on Accreditation.

AWHONN also holds a California BRN number: California CNE provider #CEP580.

Accredited status does not imply endorsement by the provider or ANCC of any commercial products displayed or discussed in conjunction with an activity.

The maximum CNE credit that can be earned while attending the Advanced Fetal Heart Monitoring Course is eight (8) AWHONN contact hours. Participants must attend the entire course and complete the feedback document in order to receive the CNE credit.

Accreditation Statement—Physicians

This activity has been planned and implemented in accordance with the accreditation requirements and policies of the Accreditation Council for Continuing Medical Education (ACCME) through the joint providership of Professional Education Services Group and the Association of Women's Health, Obstetric and Neonatal Nurses (AWHONN). Professional Education Services Group is accredited by the ACCME to provide continuing medical education for physicians.

Credit Designation Statement—Physicians

Professional Education Services Group designates this educational activity for a maximum of 6 hours of *AMA PRA Category 1 Credits*™. Physicians should claim only the credit commensurate with the extent of their participation in the activity.

DISCLAIMER

This course and all accompanying materials (publication) were developed by AWHONN, in cooperation with PESG, as an educational resource for fetal heart monitoring. It presents general methods and techniques of practice that are currently acceptable, based on current research and techniques used by recognized authorities. Proper care of individual patients may depend on many individual factors in clinical practice, as well as professional judgment in the techniques described herein. Clinical circumstances naturally vary, and professionals must use their own best judgment in accordance with the patients' needs and preferences, professional standards and institutional rules. Variations and innovations that are consistent with law, and that demonstrably improve the quality of patient care, should be encouraged.

AWHONN has sought to confirm the accuracy of the information presented herein and to describe generally accepted practices. However, AWHONN is not responsible for errors or omissions or for any consequences from application of the information in this resource and makes no warranty, expressed or implied, with respect to the contents of the publication.

Competent clinical practice depends on a broad array of personal characteristics, training, judgment, professional skills and institutional processes. This publication is simply one of many information resources. This publication is not intended to replace ongoing evaluation of knowledge and skills in the clinical setting. Nor has it been designed for use in hiring, promotion or termination decisions or in resolving legal disputes or issues of liability.

AWHONN believes that the drug selection and dosage set forth in this text are in accordance with current recommendations and practice at the time of publication. However, in view of ongoing research, changes in government regulations and the constant flow of information relating to drug therapy and drug reactions, the reader is urged to check other information available in other published sources for each drug to identify changes in indications, dosages, added warnings and precautions. This is particularly important when the recommended agent is a new or infrequently employed drug. In addition, appropriate medication use may depend on unique factors such as individuals' health status, other medication use and other factors which the professional must consider in clinical practice.

The content of this section is intended to provide information about the NICHD definitions, descriptions of electronic fetal monitoring tracing characteristics and categories of the tracings.

Additional resources include documents that are published in the *Fetal Heart Monitoring Principles and Practices 5th edition* text:

- NICHD Descriptive Terms and Categories
- Three-Tier FHR Interpretation System

The Reference listing is intended to offer participants and Instructors additional resources for review in preparation for the Advanced Fetal Monitoring Course. Many participants have found these references valuable in developing guidelines and protocols for clinical practice. AWHONN FHM Instructors should review the references to support the course teaching materials and to prepare for potential questions by their course participants.

FETAL HEART RATE CHARACTERISTICS AND PATTERNS: 2008 NICHD DESCRIPTIVE TERMS FOR FETAL HEART RATE CHARACTERISTICS

Term	Definition
Baseline Rate	Approximate mean FHR rounded to increments of 5 bpm during a 10-minute segment, excluding accelerations and decelerations and periods of marked variability. In any 10-minute window, the minimum baseline duration must be at least 2 minutes (not necessarily contiguous) or the baseline for that period is indeterminate. In this case, one may need to refer to the previous 10-minute segment for determination of the baseline.
Bradycardia	Baseline rate of <110 bpm.
Tachycardia	Baseline rate of >160 bpm.
Baseline Variability	Fluctuations in the baseline FHR are irregular in amplitude and frequency and are visually quantified as the amplitude of the peak to trough in bpm.
– Absent variability	Amplitude range undetectable.
– Minimal variability	Amplitude range visually detectable (>undetectable) but ≤5 bpm.
– Moderate variability	Amplitude range 6–25 bpm.
– Marked variability	Amplitude range >25 bpm.
Acceleration	Visually apparent *abrupt* increase (onset to peak is <30 seconds) in FHR above the adjacent baseline. The FHR peak is ≥15 bpm above the baseline and lasts ≥15 seconds but <2 minutes from the onset to return to baseline. Before 32 weeks of gestation, a peak ≥10 bpm above the baseline and duration of ≥10 seconds is an acceleration.
Prolonged Acceleration	Acceleration ≥2 minutes but <10 minutes duration.
Early Deceleration	Visually apparent, usually symmetrical *gradual* decrease (onset to nadir is ≥30 seconds) of the FHR and return to baseline associated with a uterine contraction. This decrease in FHR is calculated from the onset to the nadir of the deceleration. The nadir of deceleration occurs at the same time as the peak of the contraction. In most cases, the onset, nadir and recovery of the deceleration are coincident with the beginning, peak and ending of the contraction, respectively.

(*continued*)

Term	Definition
Late Deceleration	Visually apparent, usually symmetrical *gradual* decrease (onset to nadir is ≥30 seconds) of the FHR and return to baseline associated with a uterine contraction. This decrease is calculated from the onset to the nadir of the deceleration. It is delayed in timing, with the nadir of deceleration occurring after the peak of the contraction. In most cases, the onset, nadir and recovery of the deceleration occur after the onset, peak and ending of the contraction, respectively.
Variable Deceleration	Visually apparent *abrupt* decrease (onset to beginning of nadir is <30 seconds) in FHR below baseline. The decrease is calculated from the onset to the nadir of the deceleration. Decrease is 15 bpm, lasting ≥15 seconds but <2 minutes in duration. When variable decelerations are associated with uterine contractions, their onset, depth and duration vary with successive uterine contractions.
Prolonged Deceleration	Visually apparent decrease in FHR below baseline. Decrease is ≥15 bpm, lasting ≥2 minutes but <10 minutes from onset to return to baseline.
	A deceleration that lasts greater than or equal to 10 minutes is a baseline change.
Recurrent	Occurring with ≥50% of contractions in a 20-minute period.
Intermittent	Occurring with <50% of contractions in a 20-minute period.
Sinusoidal	Visually apparent undulating sine wave-like pattern in FHR baseline and cycle frequency of 3–5 per minute which persists for ≥20 minutes.

Macones, G. A., Hankins, G. D., Spong, C. Y., Hauth, J. D., & Moore, T. (2008). The 2008 National Institute of Child Health Human Development workshop report on electronic fetal monitoring: Update on definitions, interpretations, and research guidelines. *Obstetrics & Gynecology, 112*, 661–666; and *Journal of Obstetric, Gynecologic and Neonatal Nursing, 37*, 510–515.

2008 THREE-TIER FETAL HEART RATE INTERPRETATION SYSTEM

Category I
*Category I fetal heart rate (FHR) tracings include **all** of the following:* • Baseline rate: 110–160 beats per minute (bpm) • Baseline FHR variability: moderate • Late or variable decelerations: absent • Early decelerations: present or absent • Accelerations: present or absent

Category II
Category II FHR tracings include all FHR tracings not categorized as Category I or Category III. Category II tracings may represent an appreciable fraction of those encountered in clinical care. Examples of Category II FHR tracings include any of the following: **Baseline Rate** • Bradycardia not accompanied by baseline variability • Tachycardia **Baseline FHR Variability** • Minimal baseline variability • Absent baseline variability not accompanied by recurrent decelerations • Marked baseline variability **Accelerations** • Absence of induced accelerations after fetal stimulation **Periodic or Episodic Decelerations** • Recurrent variable decelerations accompanied by minimal or moderate baseline variability • Prolonged deceleration $\geq$ 2 minutes but $<$ 10 minutes • Recurrent late decelerations with moderate baseline variability • Variable decelerations with other characteristics, such as slow return to baseline, "overshoots," or "shoulders"

Category III

Category III FHR tracings include either
 	
• Absent baseline FHR variability and any of the following:
  - Recurrent late decelerations
  - Recurrent variable decelerations
  - Bradycardia
• Sinusoidal pattern

REFERENCES

Introduction and Oxygenation

American College of Obstetricians and Gynecologists and the American Academy of Pediatrics. (2014). Neonatal encephalopathy and neurologic outcome (2nd ed.). Washington, DC: Author.

American College of Obstetricians and Gynecologists. (2016). Practice Bulletin Premature rupture of membranes. Washington, DC: Author. Published in Obstetrics and Gynecology, 127 (1), e39–e51.

Blackburn, S. (2013). Maternal, fetal and neonatal physiology: A clinical perspective (4th ed., pp. 165–166). Maryland Heights: Elsevier Saunders.

Bobrowski, R. (2010). Pulmonary physiology in pregnancy. Clinical Obstetrics and Gynecology, 53(2), 285–300. doi: 10.1097/GRF.ob013e318e04776.

Clark, S., Belfort, M., Saade, G., Hankins, G., Miller, D., Frye, D., & Myers, J. (2007). Implementation of a conservative checklist-based protocol for oxytocin administration: Maternal and newborn outcomes. American Journal of Obstetrics and Gynecology, 197(5), 480.e1–480.e5. doi: http://dx.doi.org/10.1016/j.ajog.2007.08.026.

Clark, S., Simpson, K., Knox, E., & Garite, T. (2009) Oxytocin: New perspectives on an old drug. American Journal of Obstetrics and Gynecology, 200(1), 35.e1–35.e6. doi: http://dx.doi.org/10.1016/j.ajog.2008.06.010

Cohn, H., Sacks, E., Heyman, M., & Rudolph, A. (1974). Cardiovascular responses to hypoxemia and acidemia in fetal lambs. American Journal of Obstetrics and Gynecology, 120(6), 817–824.

Cunningham, F., Leveno, K., & Bloom, S. (2014). Williams Obstetrics. United States: McGraw Hill Medical.

King, T. (2013). Fetal assessment. In S. Blackburn (Ed.), Maternal, fetal and neonatal physiology: A clinical perspective (4th ed.). Maryland Heights: Elsevier.

King, T. & Parer, J. (2000). The physiology of fetal heart rate patterns and perinatal asphyxia. Journal of Perinatal and Neonatal Nursing, 14(3), 19–39.

Lowe, N. & Reiss, R. (1996). Parturition and fetal adaptation. Journal of Obstetric, Gynecologic and Neonatal Nursing, 25, 339-349.

Lyndon, A. & Usher-Ali, L. (Eds.), (2015). Fetal heart monitoring principles and practices (5th ed., second printing). Washington, DC: Kendall Hunt Publishing Company.

Macones, G., Hankins, G., Spong, C., Hauth, J., & Moore, T. (2008). The 2008 National Institute of Child Health Human Development workshop report on electric fetal monitoring: Update on definitions, interpretation and research guidelines. Obstetrics & Gynecology, 112, 661–666.

Mecham, C. Pulse Oximetry. In UpToDate, Waltham, MA. http://www.uptodate.com/contents/pulse-oximetry-in-adults.

Meschia. G. (1979). Supply of oxygen to the fetus. Journal of Reproductive Medicine, 23, 160–165.

Meschia. G. (2009). Placental respiratory gas exchange and fetal oxygenation. In R. Creasy, R. Resnik, J. Iams, C. Lockwood, & T. Moore, (Eds.). Creasy and Resnik's maternal Fetal medicine: Principles and practice (6th ed., pp. 181–191). Philadelphia: Saunders Elsevier.

Miller, D., Miller, L., & Cypher, R. (2017). Mosby's pocket guide to fetal monitoring: A multidisciplinary approach (8th ed.). United States: Mosby.

Nageotte, M. & Gilstrap, L. (2009). Intrapartum surveillance. In R. Creasy, R. Resnik, J. Imas, C. Lockwood, & T. Moore (Eds.), Creasy and Resnik's maternal fetal medicine: Principles and practice (6th ed., pp. 397–417). Philadelphia: Saunders Elsevier.

Parer, J. (1997). Handbook of fetal heart rate monitoring (2nd ed.). Philadelphia: Saunders Elsevier.

Price, S. & Wilson, L. (2003). Pathophysiology: Clinical concepts of disease processes (6th ed.). St. Louis: Mosby.

Simpson, K. & Creehan, P. (Eds.), (2013). Perinatal nursing (4th ed.). Philadelphia: Lippincott Williams Wilkins.

Wagner, P., Powell, F., & West. J. (2010). Ventilation, blood flow and gas exchange in Mason, R., Broaddus, V., Martin, T., King, T., Schraufnagel, D., Murray, J., & Nadel, J. (Eds.), Murray and Nadel's textbook of respiratory medicine (Vol. 1, 5th ed.). Philadelphia: Saunders Elsevier.

Fetal Arrythmias

American College of Obstetricians and Gynecologists. (2013). Practice Bulletin 115: Vaginal Trial of Labor after Cesarean Birth. Author: Washington, DC.

American Heart Association What is Arrhythmia? http://www.heart.org/HEARTORG/Conditions/Arrhythmia/AboutArrhythmia/About-Arrhythmia_UCM_002010_Article.jsp#.V-qjJ_ArKM8

Api, O. & Carvalho, J. (2008). Fetal dysrhythmias. Best Practice and Research Clinical Obstetrics and Gynecology, 22(1), 31–48.

Blackburn, S. (2013). Maternal, fetal and neonatal physiology: A clinical perspective, (4th ed.).Maryland Heights: Elsevier Saunders.

Copel, J., Liang, R., Demasio, K., Ozeren, S., & Kleinman, C. (2000). The clinical significance of the irregular fetal heart rhythm. American Journal of Obstetrics and Gynecology, 182, 813–819.

Cuneo, B. (2006). Outcome of fetal cardiac defects. Current Opinion Pediatrics, 18, 490–496.

Fineman, J. & Clyman, R. (2009). Fetal cardiovascular physiology. In R. Creasy, R. Resnik, J. Iams, C. Lockwood, & T. Moore (Eds.), Maternal-fetal medicine (6th ed.). Philadelphia: Saunders.

France, R. (2006). A review of fetal circulation and the segmental approach in fetal echocardiography. Journal of Diagnostic Medical Sonography, 2, 29–39.

Freeman, R., Garite, T., & Nageotte, M. (2003). Fetal heart monitoring (3rd ed.). Philadelphia: Lippincott, Williams & Wilkins.

Garite, T. (2007). Intrapartum fetal evaluation. In S. Gabbe, J. Niebyl, & J. Simpson (Eds.), Obstetrics: Normal and problem pregnancies (5th ed., pp. 364–395). Philadelphia: Churchill Livingstone.

Hameed, A. & Sklansky, M. (2007). Pregnancy: Maternal and fetal heart disease. Current Problems in Cardiology, 32, 419–494.

Jaeggi, E. & Friedberg, M. (2008). Diagnosis and management of fetal bradyarrhythmias. Pacing and Clinical Electrophysiology, 31(1 Suppl. 1) S50–S53. doi:10.1111/j.1540-8159.2008.00957.x

Jaeggi, E. & Nii, M. (2005). Fetal brady and tachyarrhythmias: New and accepted diagnostic and treatment methods. Seminars in Fetal and Neonatal Medicine, 10, 504–514.

Kiserud, T. (2005). Physiology of the fetal circulation. Seminars in Fetal and Neonatal Medicine, 10, 493–503.

Kleinman, C. (2006). Prenatal cardiac therapy. In M. Evans, M. Johnson, Y. Yaron, & A. Drugan (Eds.), Prenatal diagnosis (pp. 671–682). New York: McGraw-Hill.

Kleinman, C. & Nehgme, R. (2004). Cardiac arrhythmias in the human fetus. Pediatric Cardiology, 25(3), 234–251.

Larmay, H. & Strasburger, J. (2004). Differential diagnosis and management of the fetus and newborn with an irregular or abnormal heart rate. Pediatric Clinics of North America, 51(4), 1033–1050.

Luigi, D. & Walsh, E. Epidemiology, clinical manifestations, and diagnosis of the Wolff-Parkinson-White syndrome. In: S. Levy, B. Knight, & B. Downey (Eds.), UpTo-Date. Waltham, MA. http://www.uptodate.com/contents/epidemiology-clinical-manifestations-and-diagnosis-of-the-wolff-parkinson-white-syndrome.

Lyndon, A. & Usher Ali, L. (Eds.), (2015). Fetal heart monitoring principles and practices (5th ed., Second printing). Washington DC: Kendall/Hunt Publishing Company.

Macones, G. A., Hankins, G. D., Spong, C. Y., Hauth, J. D., & Moore, T. (2008). The 2008 National Institute of Child Health Human Development workshop report on electronic fetal monitoring: Update on definitions, interpretations, and research guidelines. Obstetrics and Gynecology, 112, 661–666. doi:10.1097/AOG.0b013e3181841395; and Journal of Obstetric, Gynecologic and Neonatal Nursing, 37, 510–515.

Mielke, B. & Benda, N. (2001). Cardiac output and central distribution of blood flow in the human fetus. Circulation, 103, 1662–1668.

Nageotte, M. & Gilstrap, L. (2009). Intrapartum fetal surveillance. In R. Creasy, R. Resnik, J. Iams, C. Lockwood, & T. Moore (Eds.), Maternal-fetal medicine (6th ed., pp. 398–417). Philadelphia: Saunders.

Oudijk, M., Michon, M., Kleinman, C., Kapusta, L., Stoutenbeek, Pl, Visser, G., et al. (2000). Sotalol to treat fetal dysrhythmias. Circulation, 101, 2721–2726.

Parker, L. (2006). Hydrops fetalis. Newborn and Infant Nursing Reviews, 6, e1–e8.

Pedra, S., Smallhorn, J., Ryan, G., Chitayat, D., Taylor, G. Khan, R., et al. (2002). Fetal cardiomyopoathies: Pathogenic mechanisms, hemodynamic findings and clinical outcome. Circulation, 106, 585–591.

Rychik, J. (2006). Fetal cardiovascular physiology. Pediatric Cardiology, 25, 201–209.

Simpson, J. & Sharland, G. (1998). Fetal tachycardias: Management and outcome of 127 consecutive cases. Heart, 79, 576–578.

Strasburger, J. (2000). Fetal arrhythmias. Progress in Pediatric Cardiology, 11 (1), 1–17.

Strasburger, J., Cheulkar, B., & Wichman, H. (2007). Perinatal arrhythmias: Diagnosis and management. Clinics in Perinatology, 34(4), 627–652, vii–viii.

Wren, Cl. (2006). Cardiac arrhythmias in the fetus and newborn. Seminars in Fetal and Neonatal Medicine, 11(3), 182–190.

Complex Case Studies

American College of Obstetricians and Gynecologists and the American Academy of Pediatrics (2014). Neonatal encephalopathy and neurologic outcome (2nd ed.). Washington, DC: Author.

American College of Obstetricians and Gynecologist. (2013). Task force on hypertension in pregnancy. Washington, DC: author.

American College of Obstetricians and Gynecologist. (2000, Reaffirmed 2016). Practice Bulletin Number 161, External cephalic version. Obstetrics and Gynecology, 127, e54–e61.

Beloosesky, R. & Ross, M. (2016). Polyhydramnios. In C. J. Lockwood, D. Levine, & V. A. Barss (Eds.), Uptodate. Waltman, MA. http://www.uptodate.com/contents/polyhydramnios?source=machineLearning&search=polyhydramnios&selectedTitle=1%7E108&sectionRank=4&anchor=H350993446#H350993446

Collins, P., Lilley, G., Bruynseels, D., Burkett-St. Laurent, D., Cannings-John, R., Precious, E., et al. (2014). Fibrin-based clot formation as an early and rapid biomarker for progression of postpartum hemorrhage: a prospective study. Blood 124, 1727–1736. doi:10.1182/blood-2014-04-567891

Cunningham, G., Leveno, K., Bloom, S., Spong, C., Dashe, J., Hoffman, B., et al. (2014). Williams obstetrics (24th ed.). United States: McGraw-Hill Medical.

Greenwell, E., Wyshak G., Ringer S., Johnson, L., Rivkin, M., & Lieberman, E. (2012) Intrapartum temperature elevation, epidural use, and adverse outcome in term infants. Pediatrics 129, e447–e454.

Impey, L., Greenwood, C., Black, R., Yeh, P., Sheil, O., &, Doyle, P. (2008). The relationship between intrapartum maternal fever and neonatal acidosis as risk factors for neonatal encephalopathy. American Journal of Obstetrics and Gynecology 198, 49.el–49.e6.

Jeejeebhoy F., Zelop C., Lipman S., Carvalho, B., Joglar, J., Mhyre J., et al. (2015). On behalf of the American Heart Association Emergency Cardiovascular Care Committee, Council on Cardiopulmonary, Critical Care, Perioperative and Resuscitation, Council on Cardiovascular Diseases in the Young, and Council on Clinical Cardiology. Cardiac arrest in pregnancy: A scientific statement from the American Heart Association. Circulation, 132, 1747–1773.

Leung, A., Leung, E., & Paul, R. (1993). Uterine rupture after previous cesarean delivery: maternal and fetal consequences. American Journal of Obstetrics and Gynecology, 169, 945–950.

Lyndon, A., & Usher Ali, L. (Eds.), (2015). Fetal heart monitoring principles and practices (5th ed., second printing). Washington DC: Kendall/Hunt Publishing Company.

Macones, G., Hankins, G., Spong, C., Hauth, J., & Moore, T. (2008). The 2008 National Institute of Child Health Human Development workshop report on electronic fetal monitoring: Update on definitions, interpretations, and research guidelines. Obstetrics and Gynecology, 112, 661–666. doi:10.1097/AOG.0b013e3181841395; and Journal of Obstetric, Gynecologic and Neonatal Nursing, 37, 510–515.

Modanlou, H. & Murata, Y. (2004). Sinusoidal heart rate pattern: Reappraisal of its definition and clinical significance. Journal of Obstetrics and Gynaecology Research, 30, 169–180.

Reddy , A., Moulden, M., & redman, C. (2009). Antepartum high-frequency fetal heart rate sinusoidal rhythm: Computerized detection and fetal anemia. American Journal of Obstetrics and Gynecology, 200(4), 407.el-407.e6.doi:10:1016/j.ajog.2008.10.026

Smith, J. F., & Wax, J.R. (2015). Rupture of the unscarred uterus. In C. J. Lockwood, & V. A. Barss (Eds.), Uptodate. Waltman, MA. Retrieved http://www.uptodate.com/contents/rupture-of-the-unscarred-uterus?source=machineLearning&search=uterine+rupture&selectedTitle=2%7E120&sectionRank=2&anchor=H122632318#H122632318

Victory, R., Penava, D., Da Silva, O., Natale, R., & Richardson, B. (2004). Umbilical cord pH and base excess values in relation to adverse outcome events for infants delivering at term. American Journal of Obstetrics and Gynecology, 191 (6), 2021–2028.

Teamwork, Communication, and Documentation

Afors, K. & Chandraharan, E. (2011). Use of Continuous Electronic Fetal Monitoring in a Preterm Fetus: Clinical Dilemmas and Recommendations for Practice. Journal of Pregnancy. doi:10.1155/2011/848794. Volume 2011, Article ID 848794. 7 pages (no range indicated in citation directions)

Agency for Healthcare Research and Quality. (2007). Team STEPPS© Curriculum. Rockville, MD: Author.

American Academy of Pediatrics and American College of Obstetricians and Gynecologists. (2012). Guidelines for perinatal care (7th ed.). Elk Grove Village, IL: Author.

American Association of Critical-Care Nurses. (2005). AACN standards for establishing and sustaining healthy work environments. Aliso Viejo, CA: Author.

American College of Obstetricians and Gynecologists. (2000). Operative vaginal delivery, (Practice Bulletin Number 17). Washington, DC: Author.

American College of Obstetricians and Gynecologists. (2009a). Informed consent, (Committee Opinion Number 439). Washington, DC: Author.

American College of Obstetricians and Gynecologists. (2009b). Induction of labor (Practice Bulletin Number 107). Washington, DC: Author.

American College of Obstetricians and Gynecologists. (2010). Vaginal birth after previous cesarean delivery. Washington, DC: Author.

American College of Obstetricians and Gynecologists Committee on Patient Safety and Quality Improvement. (2011a). Disruptive behavior, (Committee Opinion Number 508). Washington, DC: Author.

American College of Obstetricians and Gynecologists. (2011b). Preoperative planned cesarean delivery (Patient Safety Checklist Number 4). Washington, DC: Author. doi:10.1097/AOG.0b013e3182ed223

American College of Obstetricians and Gynecologists Committee on Patient Safety and Quality Improvement. (2011c). Partnering with patients to improve safety (Committee Opinion Number 490). Washington, DC: Author.

American College of Obstetricians and Gynecologists Task Force on Hypertension in Pregnancy. (2013). Hypertension in pregnancy. Washington, DC: Author.

American Nurses Association. (2010). ANA's principles for nursing documentation. Retrieved from http://www.nursesbooks.org/Main-Menu/Specialties/Staffing-Workplace/eBook-Principles-for-Nursing-Documentation.aspx

Association of Women's Health, Obstetric and Neonatal Nurses. (2008). Nursing management of the second stage of labor. Evidence-based clinical practice guideline. Washington, DC: Author.

Association of Women's Health, Obstetric and Neonatal Nurses. (2015). Fetal Heart Monitoring Position Statement. Washington, DC: Author.

Baird, S. & Ruth, D. (2002). Electronic Fetal Monitoring of the Preterm Fetus. Journal of Perinatal and Neonatal Nursing. 16(1), 12–24.

Centers for Disease Control and Prevention (2010). Prevention of perinatal group B streptococcal disease: Revised guidelines from CDC, 2010. Morbidity and Mortality Weekly Report, 19(RR-10), 1–36.

Cunningham, F., Leveno, K., Bloom, S., Spong, C., Dashe, J., Hoffman, B., et al. (2014). Williams obstetrics, (24th ed.). New York: McGraw-Hill.

Deshpande, N. & Oxford, C. (2012). Management of pregnant patients who refuse medically indicated cesarean delivery. Reviews in Obstetrics and Gynecology, 5(3/4), 144–150.

Glantz, J. & Bertoia, N. (2011). Preterm nonstress testing: 10-beat compared with 15-beat criteria. Obstetrics and Gynecology, 118(1), 87–93.

Griffin, T. (2010). Bringing change of shift report to the bedside. Journal of Perinatal and Neonatal Nursing, 24(4), 338–353.

Jacobson, C., Zlatnik, M., Kennedy, H., & Lyndon, A. (2013). Nurses' perspectives on the intersection of safety and informed decision making in maternity care. Journal of Obstetric, Gynecologic and Neonatal Nursing, 42(5), 577–587.

Lyndon, A., Sexton, B., Simpson, K.R., Rosenstein, A., Lee, K., & Wachter, R. (2012). Predictors of likelihood of speaking up about safety concerns in labour and delivery. BMJ Quality and Safety, 21(9), 791–799. doi:10.1136/bmqs.2010.050211

Lyndon, A. & Usher Ali, L. (Eds.), (2015). Fetal heart monitoring principles and practices, (5th ed., Print book). Washington DC: Kendall/Hunt Publishing Company.

Macones, G., Hankins, G., Spong, C., Hauth, J., & Moore, T. (2008). The 2008 National Institute of Child Health and Human Development workshop report on electronic fetal Monitoring: Update on definitions, interpretations, and research guidelines. Obstetrics and Gynecology, 112, 661–666; and Journal of Obstetric, Gynecologic and Neonatal Nursing, 37, 510-515.

Prielipp, R. , Magro, M., Morell, R., & Brull, S. (2010). The normalization of deviance: Do we unknowingly accept doing the wrong thing? AANA Journal, 78(4), 284–287.

Simpson, K. (2005). Handling handoffs safely. MCN: The American Journal of Maternal/Child Nursing, 30(2), 152.

Simpson, K. (2014). Perinatal patient safety and professional liability issues. In K. R. Simpson & P. A. Creehan (Eds.), Perinatal nursing (4th ed., pp. 1–40). Philadelphia, Pad: Lippincott Williams & Wilkins.

The Joint Commission. (2008). Behaviors that undermine a culture of safety. Sentinel Event Alert, 40, 1–3. Retrieved from http://www.jointcommission.org/sentinel_event_alert_issue_40_behaviors_that_undermine_a_culture_of_safety/

True, B., Cochrane, C., Sleutel, M., Newcomb, P., Tullar, P., & Sammons Jr., J. (2016). Developing and testing a vaginal delivery safety checklist. Journal of Obstetric, Gynecologic and Neonatal Nursing, 45, 239–248. doi: http://dx.doi.org/10.1016/j.jogn.2015.12.010.

Woodward, P., Kennedy, A., Sohaey, R., Byrne, J., Oh, K., Puchalski, M., et al. (2011). Diagnostic imaging: Obstetrics (2nd ed.). Salt Lake City, UT: Amirsys.

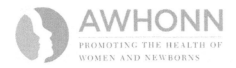

AWHONN
PROMOTING THE HEALTH OF
WOMEN AND NEWBORNS

The Association of Women's Health, Obstetric and Neonatal Nurses (AWHONN) is the leading professional association committed to promoting the health of women and newborns. AWHONN provides the tools and resources to help you become a great nurse! By joining AWHONN you open the door to a wealth of educational resources and opportunities to help you take the next step in your personal and professional development.

Membership Benefits

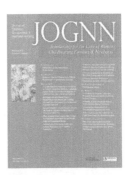

- Subscription to *Journal of Obstetric, Gynecologic and Neonatal Nursing* (JOGNN)
- Subscription to *Nursing for Women's Health*
- Access to Free Webinars and Journal CNE through the AWHONN Online Learning Center
- Free member-only tools and resources
- AWHONN's bi-weekly *SmartBrief* email newsletter
- Discounts on Annual Convention Registration
- Networking & Peer Education Opportunities through Local Sections & Chapters
- Professional Development and Leadership Opportunities
- Access to Career Management Tools in the AWHONN Career Center
- Special discounts on Personal Liability & Auto Insurance, Scrubs, Travel, Car Rental, Financial Planning, and more!

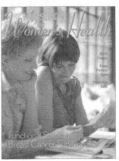

Visit www.awhonn.org to join and start taking advantage of your member benefits today!

AWHONN Advanced Fetal Monitoring Course

1

About AWHONN

The Association of Women's Health, Obstetric and Neonatal Nurses (AWHONN) is the foremost nursing authority promoting the health of women and newborns and strengthening the nursing profession through the delivery of advocacy, research, education and evidence-based clinical resources.

AWHONN represents the interests of 350,000 registered nurses working in women's health, obstetric and neonatal nurses across the United States.

2

Key Activities

- Two Leading Scholarly Journals:
  - *JOGNN/Nursing for Women's Health*
- Annual Convention
- Fetal Heart Monitoring Program
- Advocacy Work and Research Program
- Evidence-Based Clinical Practice Guidelines
- Webinars and Online Education

3

Disclosures

The Instructors presenting this course will report either conflicts of interest or relevant financial relationships, or lack thereof.

The nurse planners for this course report no significant financial or other relationships with commercial entities.

4

Course Objectives

- Describe physiologic principles of maternal and fetal oxygen transfer as they apply to principles of fetal heart monitoring.

- Recognize fetal cardiac arrhythmia patterns and describe potential outcomes associated with these patterns.

5

Course Objectives

- Analyze complex case studies and tracings utilizing standardized terminology.

- Apply perinatal risk management principles, communication techniques and documentation strategies to complex and challenging patient care scenarios.

6

Fetal Oxygenation

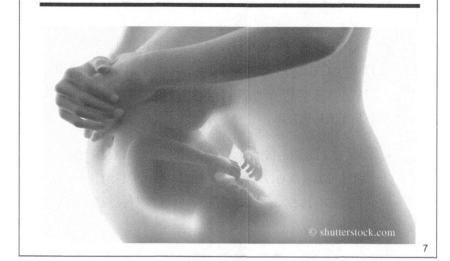

© shutterstock.com

7

Maternal Oxygenation System

- Animation of oxygenation

8

Maternal Transfer of Oxygen to Fetus

Atmosphere to alveoli

↓

Diffusion across alveolar membrane

↓

Lungs to placenta

↓

Diffusion across placenta

Adapted from Meschia, G. (1979). Supply of oxygen to the fetus. *Journal Reproductive Medicine*, 23, 160.

9

_____

_____

_____

_____

Maternal Transfer of Oxygen to Fetus

Transport from placenta to fetus

Diffusion into fetal tissues

Adapted from Meschia, G. (1979). Supply of oxygen to the fetus. *Journal Reproductive Medicine*, 23, 160.

10

_____

_____

_____

_____

Components of Oxygen Transport

- Oxygen content

- Oxygen affinity

- Oxygen delivery

- Oxygen consumption

11

Maternal Oxygen Content

Total amount of oxygen in arterial blood:

- Amount of oxygen dissolved in plasma
  – Partial pressure of oxygen—PaO_2

- Oxygen saturation
  – % of oxygen carried on hemoglobin—SaO_2

12

Partial Pressure of Oxygen

Partial pressure of oxygen or "oxygen tension" (PaO_2):

- Oxygen dissolved in plasma
  - 1–2% of total oxygen content

- This pressure helps bind oxygen molecules to the hemoglobin and has role in hemoglobin's *affinity for oxygen*

13

Hemoglobin Molecule

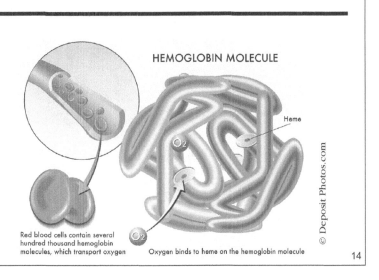

HEMOGLOBIN MOLECULE

Heme

O_2

O_2

Red blood cells contain several hundred thousand hemoglobin molecules, which transport oxygen

Oxygen binds to heme on the hemoglobin molecule

© Deposit Photos.com

14

Oxygen Saturation

Oxygen saturation (SaO_2):

- 98–99% of oxygen content is bound to hemoglobin molecules in the red blood cells

- Hemoglobin carrying four molecules of O_2 is 100% saturated

15

Pulse Oximetry

- Important points
- Implications for care

16

Oxyhemoglobin

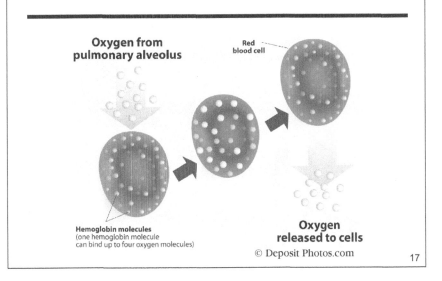

Oxygen from pulmonary alveolus

Red blood cell

Hemoglobin molecules
(one hemoglobin molecule
can bind up to four oxygen molecules)

Oxygen released to cells

© Deposit Photos.com

17

Oxygen Affinity

- The ability of hemoglobin to acquire and release oxygen molecules
- The higher PaO_2 levels in the lungs increase hemoglobin's affinity for oxygen so oxygen and hemoglobin bind
- At lower PaO_2 levels, the "affinity" is decreased and the oxygen is released from the hemoglobin

18

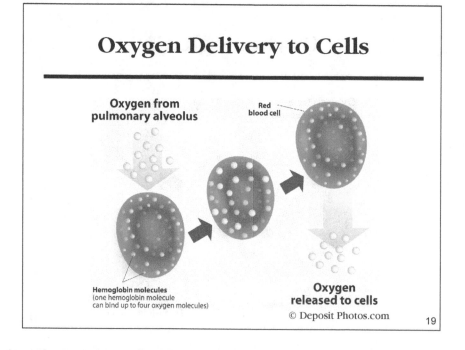

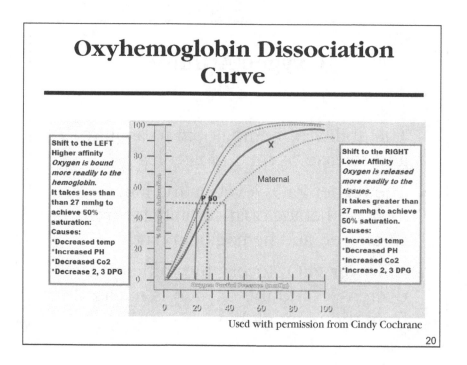

Oxyhemoglobin Dissociation Curve

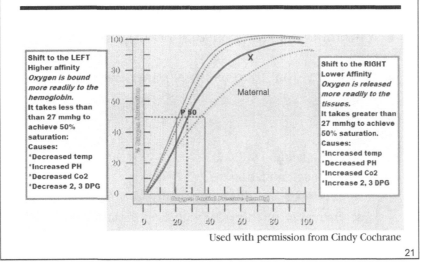

Shift to the LEFT
Higher affinity
Oxygen is bound more readily to the hemoglobin.
It takes less than than 27 mmhg to achieve 50% saturation:
Causes:
*Decreased temp
*Increased PH
*Decreased Co2
*Decrease 2, 3 DPG

Shift to the RIGHT
Lower Affinity
Oxygen is released more readily to the tissues.
It takes greater than 27 mmhg to achieve 50% saturation.
Causes:
*Increased temp
*Decreased PH
*Increased Co2
*Increase 2, 3 DPG

Used with permission from Cindy Cochrane

21

Maternal Oxygen Delivery

- Oxygen delivery is the amount of oxygen delivered to the tissues each minute
  - Two components:
    - Oxygen content:
      - ✓ Physiologic anemia of pregnancy
    - Cardiac output:
      - ✓ Increases 50% by the third trimester
      - ✓ Increases additional 20% in labor

22

Maternal Oxygen Consumption

- Amount of oxygen consumption by tissues each minute
- Conditions that increase oxygen consumption:
  - Exercise
  - Stress
  - Fever
  - Tissue healing
  - Pregnancy and labor:
    - Increases 20% during pregnancy
    - Increases another 10% with twin gestation
    - Increases another 40–60% in labor

23

Interventions to Decrease Maternal Oxygen Consumption

- Promote maternal relaxation
- Coach with helpful breathing techniques
- Manage pain
- Maintain acceptable uterine activity
- Use antipyretics to reduce fever
- Reposition the mother
- Provide appropriate management of second stage labor

24

Uterine
Oxygen Pathway/Oxygen Delivery

- Uterine arteries go through the uterine muscle wall before blood enters into the intervillous space of the placenta

- Maternal spiral arteries have decreased ability to constrict or "auto-regulate"

- Interventions to maximize uterine blood flow

25

Oxygenation: Maternal

	Oxygen Pathway	Oxygen transport Components		Potential Oxygenation Disruptions
Maternal	Maternal Lungs	Oxygen Content	Oxygen Consumption	• Upper airway obstructions • Pulmonary edema, embolus, asthma, pneumonia; ARDS • Respiratory depression
	Maternal Blood	Oxygen Content and Affinity		• Anemia
	Maternal Heart and Vasculature	Oxygen Delivery		• Hypovolemia • Regional anesthesia • Reduced cardiac output • Arrhythmia • Structural cardiac disease • Vena Cava compression
	Uterus	Oxygen Delivery		• Excessive uterine activity • Uterine Rupture

26

Placental
Oxygen Pathway/Oxygen Delivery

- Maternal side → Intervillous space → Fetal side
  - ➤ Exchange of gases, nutrients, wastes, antibodies, hormones, and some medications occurs
- Fetal reserve:
  - ➤ Placental transfer capacity
    - At 100%, the fetus has approximately twice the amount of resources it needs for growth and oxygenation
    - At less than 75%, fetal resources are limited and FGR may develop
    - At ~50% of maximal transfer, oxygen and carbon dioxide transfer decrease and the fetus can become compromised

27

Oxygen Transfer During
Contractions

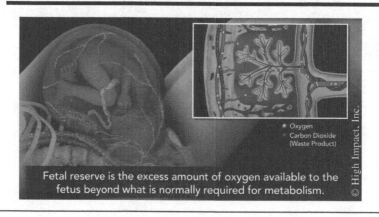

- Oxygen
- Carbon Dioxide (Waste Product)

© High Impact, Inc.

Fetal reserve is the excess amount of oxygen available to the fetus beyond what is normally required for metabolism.

28

Umbilical Cord
Oxygen Pathway/Oxygen Delivery

- Umbilical vein carries oxygen-rich blood from the placenta to the fetus

- Two umbilical arteries return deoxygenated blood from fetus back to the placenta

- Wharton's jelly helps protect the umbilical cord from compression

29

Oxygenation: Placenta and Umbilical Cord

	Oxygen Pathway	Oxygen Transport Components		Potential Oxygenation Disruptions
Placenta and Umbilical Cord	Placenta	Oxygen delivery	Oxygen Consumption	• Placental abruption • Vasa previa • Fetal maternal hemorrhage • Placental infarction • Infection
	Cord	Oxygen Delivery		• Cord compression • Cord prolapse • True knot • Abnormality in number of vessels, length, coiling and insertion.

30

Fetal Oxygen Transport: Content, Affinity, and Delivery

- Content:
  - ➤ Fetal PaO_2 is approximately 30 mmHg
- Affinity:
  - ➤ Fetal blood has higher concentration of hemoglobin and higher affinity for oxygen than maternal blood
- Delivery:
  - ➤ Fetal circulation preferentially shifts higher concentrations of oxygen to the organs that consume the most
  - ➤ Fetus has higher heart rate and cardiac output relative to its body size compared to the adult

31

Fetal Oxygen Transport: Consumption

- Fetal aerobic metabolism maintained until available oxygen in intervillous space decreases to 50% of normal levels
- The normoxic fetus compensates when experiencing transient hypoxemia:
  - ➤ Redistributes blood flow to favor the brain, heart and adrenal glands
  - ➤ Decreases total oxygen consumption:
    - As FHR slows in response to hypoxia, myocardium consumes less oxygen
    - With moderate hypoxia, fetal oxygen consumption drops to 50% of normal level
- Moves from aerobic to anaerobic metabolism

32

Fetal Adaptive Mechanism

- Oxygen binding capacity

- Shunts

- Use of oxygen

33

Aerobic Metabolism

- Requires oxygen and glucose

- Some glucose stored as glycogen

- Energy produced to be used for activity and growth

- Produces waste products:
  - Carbon dioxide
  - Water

34

Anaerobic Metabolism

- Glucose available
- Oxygen not available
- Energy produced is less than energy produced during aerobic metabolism
- Waste product produced:
  - Lactic acid:
    - Crosses placenta
    - Accumulates in fetus

35

Fetal Oxygen Consumption Maternal Pyrexia

- Studies suggest mild pyrexia during labor has an adverse impact on fetuses exposed to hypoxia ischemia, increasing later risk of encephalopathy

- Treatment goals:
  - Screen for maternal infection
  - Lower maternal temperature

36

Oxygenation: Fetal

	Oxygen Pathway	Oxygen Transport Components	Potential Oxygenation Disruptions
Fetal	Fetal blood and circulation	• Oxygen content • Oxygen affinity • Oxygen Delivery • Oxygen Consumption	• Any oxygen interruption in the maternal fetal pathway • Fetal anemia • Cardiac arrhythmia • Cardiac structural defects • Chromosomal anomaly • Infection • Twin to twin transfusion

37

Maternal—Fetal Oxygen Pathway

No Significant Interruption in Oxygen Pathway

Delivery Oxygenated infant

• As evidenced by

- Assessment

- Apgar Scores

- Cord blood gases

Significant Interruption in Oxygen Pathway

Fetal Hypoxemia
• ↓ O_2 in the blood

Fetal Hypoxia
• ↓ O_2 in the tissue

Fetal Metabolic Acidosis
• Accumulation of lactic acid in the tissue

Fetal Acidemia
• Accumulation of lactic acid in the blood

Asphyxia
• A marked impairment of gas exchange leading, if prolonged, to progressive hypoxemia, hypercapnia, and significant metabolic acidosis

Aerobic Metabolism

Converts to Anaerobic Metabolism

Delivery Infant with Possible Hypoxic Ischemic Encephalopathy

38

Work by ACOG and AAP

- 2003—ACOG published a paper about neonatal encephalopathy and cerebral palsy

- Identified criteria to define acute intrapartum hypoxic event

- 2014—released a second publication

39

Hypoxic-Ischemic Encephalopathy

- Hypoxic-ischemic encephalopathy (HIE):
  ➤ Reduced amount of oxygen and inadequate volume of blood delivered to tissues; can cause brain injury if delivery of oxygen and glucose falls below critical levels
- HIE is a subtype of neonatal encephalopathy
  ➤ Etiology is considered to be limitation of oxygen and blood flow near time of birth

ACOG and AAP (2014)

40

HIE and Cerebral Palsy

- Not all neurologic outcomes end in cerebral palsy

- Not all cerebral palsies are caused by neonatal encephalopathy

- Not all cases of neonatal encephalopathy are caused by HIE

41

Neonatal Encephalopathy: Assessment

I. Must meet case definition

II. Neonatal signs consistent with acute peripartum or intrapartum event

III. Type and timing of contributing factors are consistent with acute peripartum or intrapartum event

IV. Developmental outcomes are spastic quadriplegia or dyskinetic cerebral palsy

42

Neonatal Encephalopathy: I. Case definition

"A clinically defined syndrome of disturbed neurologic function in the earliest days of life in an infant born at or beyond 35 weeks of gestation manifested by a subnormal level of consciousness or seizures, and often accompanied by difficulty with initiating and maintain respiration and depression of tone and reflexes."

-ACOG and AAP (2014)

43

Neonatal Encephalopathy: II. Neonatal Signs Consistent with Acute Peripartum/Intrapartum Event

A. Apgar score < 5 at 5 and 10 minutes

B. Fetal umbilical artery acidemia
   ➢ pH < 7 or base deficit ≥ 12 mmol/L or both

-ACOG and AAP (2014)

44

Neonatal Encephalopathy:
II. Neonatal Signs Consistent with Acute Peripartum/Intrapartum Event

C. Neuroimaging evidence of acute brain injury consistent with hypoxic-ischemia
  ➢ Brain MRI or Magnetic Resonance Spectroscopy

D. Presence of multisystem organ failure consistent with HIE

–ACOG and AAP (2014)

45

Neonatal Encephalopathy:
III. Type and Timing of Contributing Factors Consistent with Acute Peripartum/Intrapartum Event

A. A sentinel hypoxic or ischemic event occurring immediately before or during labor and delivery:
  ➢ Ruptured uterus
  ➢ Severe abruptio placentae
  ➢ Umbilical cord prolapse
  ➢ Amniotic fluid embolus with coincident severe and prolonged maternal hypotension and hypoxemia
  ➢ Maternal cardiovascular collapse
  ➢ Fetal exsanguination from either vasa previa or massive fetomaternal hemorrhage

–ACOG and AAP (2014)

46

Neonatal Encephalopathy:
III. Type and Timing of Contributing
Factors Consistent with Acute
Peripartum/Intrapartum Event

B. Fetal heart rate patterns consistent with acute peripartum/intrapartum events:
  ➤ Patient presenting with Category I FHR pattern that converts to Category III is suggestive of HIE
  ➤ Other FHR patterns that develop after an initial Category I FHR pattern may suggest intrapartum timing of HIE:
    ■ Tachycardia with recurrent decelerations
    ■ Persistent minimal variability with recurrent decelerations

-ACOG and AAP (2014)

47

Neonatal Encephalopathy:
III. Type and Timing of Contributing
Factors Consistent with Acute
Peripartum/Intrapartum Event

C. Timing and type of brain injury patterns based on image studies consistent with etiology of acute peripartum or intrapartum event:
  ➤ 2 MRI or magnetic resonance spectroscopy scans needed:
    ■ 24 and 96 hours of life evaluates timing of the injury
    ■ Day 10 of life or later delineates the nature and extent of cerebral injury
  ➤ Brain injury patterns via MRI typical of HIE cerebral injury:
    ■ Deep nuclear gray matter
    ■ Watershed cortical injury

48

Neonatal Encephalopathy:
III. Type and Timing of Contributing Factors Consistent with acute Peripartum/Intrapartum Events

D. No evidence of other proximal or distal factors that could be contributing factors:

➢ In presence of other significant risk factors an acute intrapartum event as sole underlying pathogenesis of neonatal encephalopathy is less likely

–ACOG and AAP (2014)

49

Neonatal Encephalopathy
IV. Developmental Outcomes

- Spastic quadriplegia

- Dyskinetic cerebral palsy:

➢ Other subtypes of CP are less likely to be associated with acute intrapartum HIE

➢ Other developmental abnormalities may occur, but are not specific to acute intrapartum HIE encephalopathy and may have other causes

–ACOG and AAP (2014)

50

NICHD FHR Interpretation System

Normal Fetal Acid-Base Status: Well-Oxygenated Fetus

All of the following:
• Baseline rate: 110-160 bpm
• Baseline variability: moderate
• Late or variable decelerations: absent
• Early decelerations: present or absent
• Accelerations: present or absent

Indeterminate: Compensatory Response

Examples:
• Moderate variability with recurrent late or variable decelerations
• Minimal variability with recurrent variable decelerations
• Absent variability without recurrent decelerations
• Bradycardia with moderate variability
• Prolonged decelerations
• Tachycardia

Abnormal Fetal Acid-Base Status

Either:
• Absent variability with:
—Recurrent late decelerations, or
—Recurrent variable decelerations, or
—Bradycardia
Or
• Sinusoidal pattern

Category I   *Category II*   *Category III*

51

Absence of Metabolic Acidemia

2200 Toco/US

52

Absence of Metabolic Acidemia

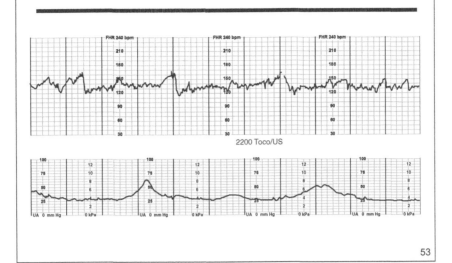

2200 Toco/US

53

Audra

- 24 years old
- $G_1 P_0$
- 40 2/7 weeks gestation
- Pregnancy course:
  - ➤ Normal prenatal labs
  - ➤ Began prenatal care @ 16 weeks
  - ➤ No complications with pregnancy

54

Audra

- Psychosocial factors
  - Married, homemaker
- Family and medical histories
  - Negative for acute and chronic illnesses

55

Audra: Admission

- SROM @ 0500, clear fluid
- Exam @ 1000:
  - No bleeding
  - 1 cm/ 60%/ −3; cephalic presentation; soft cervix
  - Abdomen
    - Soft, non-tender, no contractions
    - EFW 8½ lbs.

56

Audra: Admission

- Audra's vital signs are
  - ➤ Temperature 97.3° F, BP 125/64, pulse 105 bpm, RR 20/min
- Weight 200 lbs., height 5'5"
- BMI 33.3-obese range
- Laboratory studies normal

57

Audra: Admission

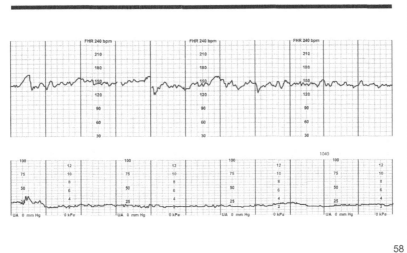

58

Audra: Admission

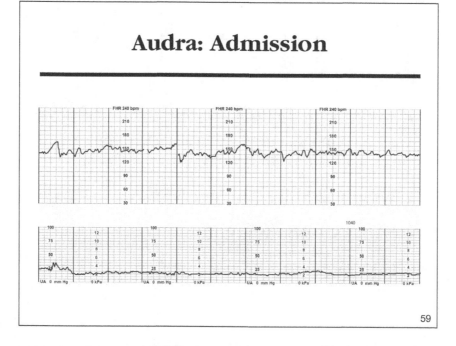

59

Audra: 20 Hours After Admission

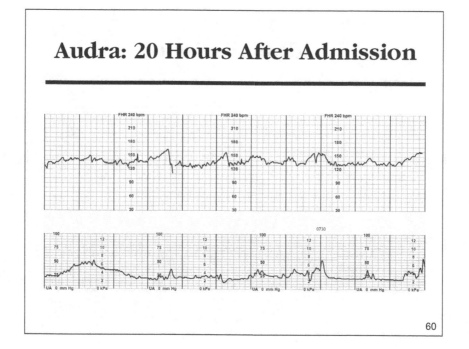

60

Audra: 1300

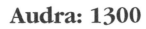

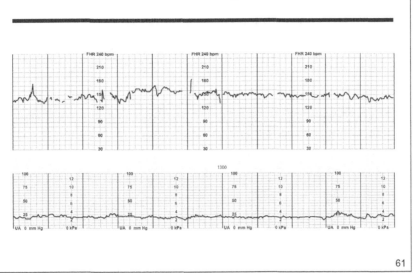

61

_____

_____

_____

_____

Audra : 1810

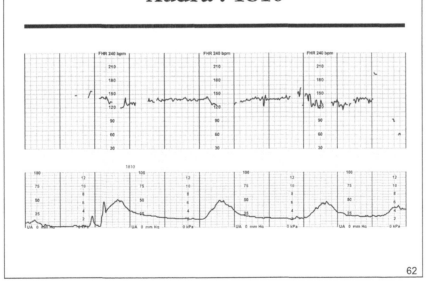

62

_____

_____

_____

_____

Audra: 2050

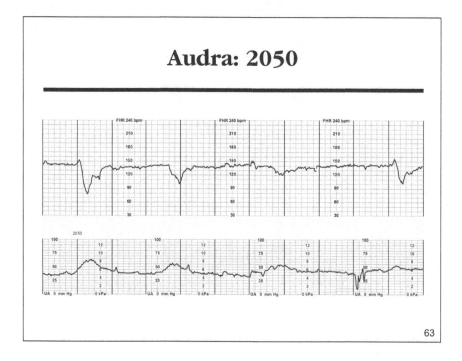

63

Audra: 2050

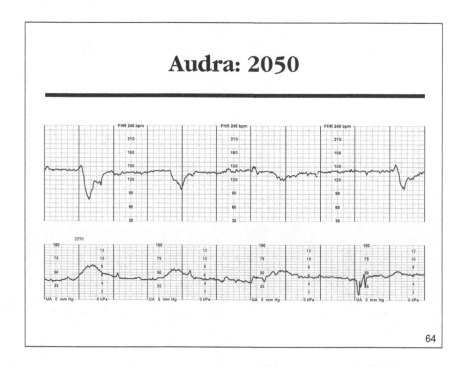

64

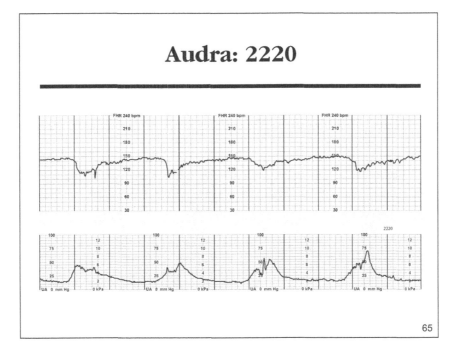

Audra: 2220

65

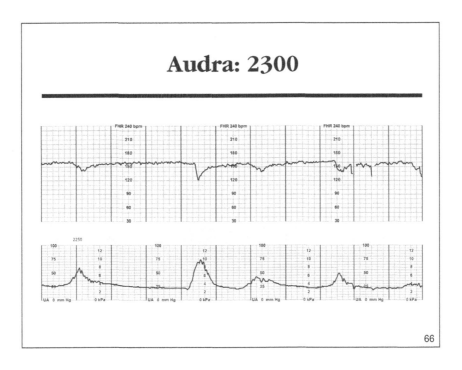

Audra: 2300

66

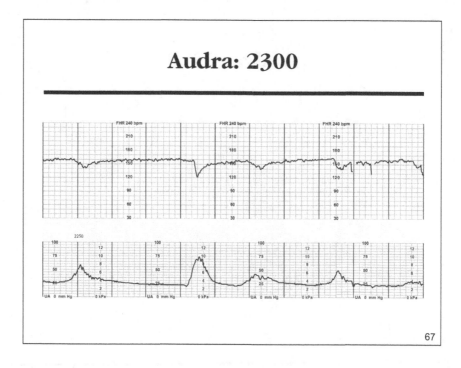

67

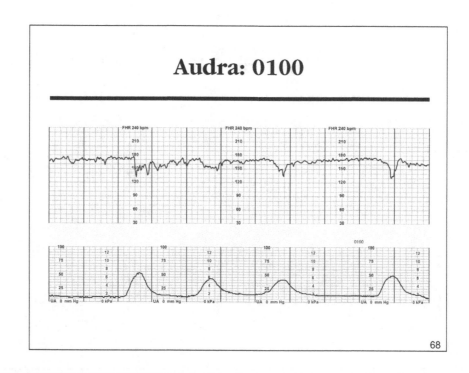

68

Audra: 0100

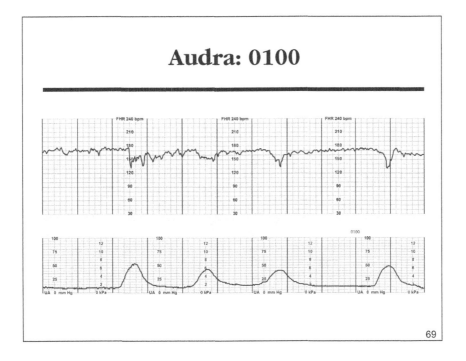

Audra: 0320

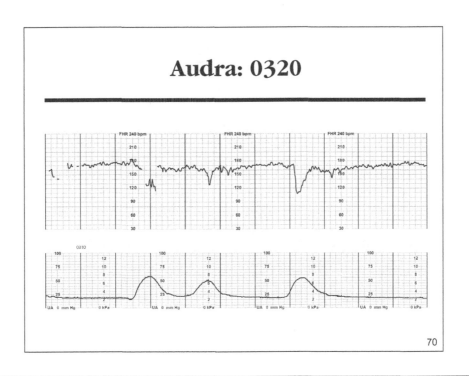

Audra: 0600

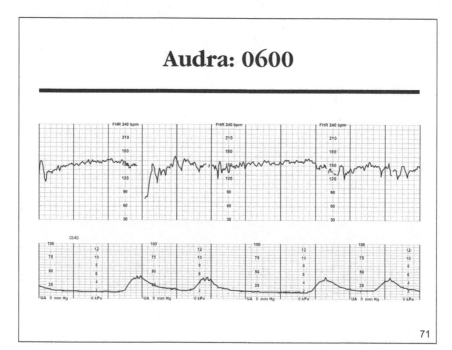

71

Audra: 0700

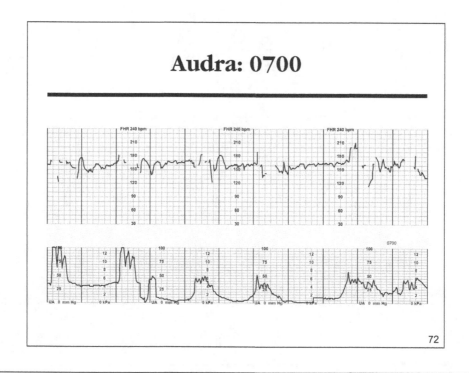

72

Audra: 0700

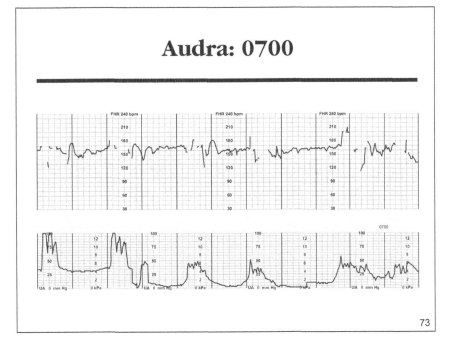

73

Audra: 0725–0739

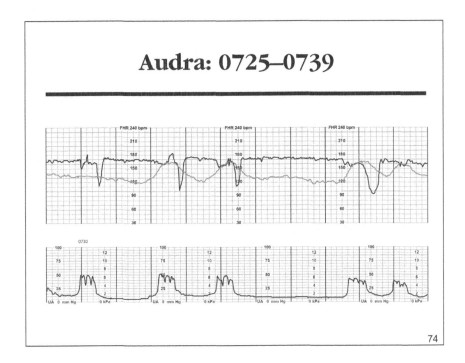

74

Audra: 0740–0754

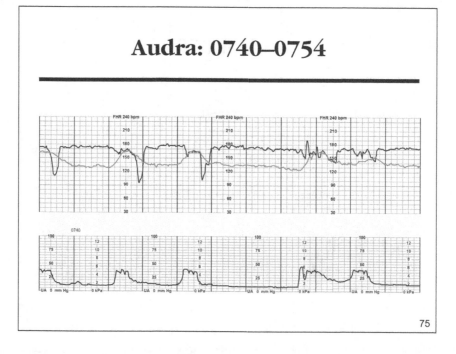

75

Audra: 0755–0801

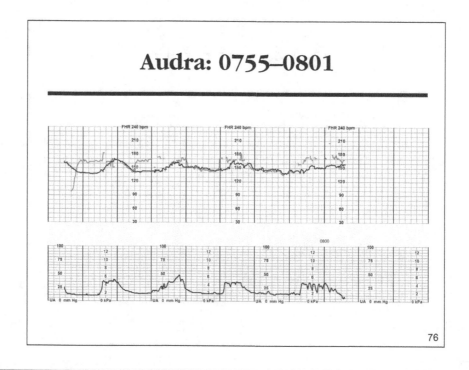

76

Audra: Delivery

- Male infant with no respiratory effort at delivery
- Apgar scores 1 and 7 at 1 and 5 minutes, respectively
- Care:
  - Tracheal suctioning, PPV, CPAP
  - To NICU

77

Audra: Delivery

- Umbilical arterial cord gases:
  - pH 6.94
  - pCO_2 92
  - pO_2 16
  - HCO_3 19.9
  - Base excess −12

78

Audra: Infant's Outcome

- Infant transferred to a children's hospital for total body cooling.

- Rewarmed 3 days later

- No seizures noted

- All cultures negative

- No evidence of cerebral palsy

79

Evaluation

- Was there evidence of oxygenation interruption?

- What markers identified by the Task Force on Neonatal Encephalopathy and Cerebral Palsy were present in Audra's case?

80

Evaluation

- Was there evidence of oxygenation interruption?

- What markers identified by the Task Force on Neonatal Encephalopathy and Cerebral Palsy were present in Audra's case?

81

Fetal Cardiac Arrhythmias

82

Cardiac Arrhythmia

- Irregular heart rhythm:
  - ➤ Falls into two broad categories:
    - Variation in the **R–R** intervals
    - Normal **P-QRS** relationship but rates fall outside of normal ranges
  - ➤ Disordered impulse formation, conduction, or both
    - Abnormal **P-QRS** relationship

83

Fetal Cardiac Arrhythmias and EFM

- Neither auscultation nor EFM alone can diagnose FHR arrhythmia

- May be noted during screening
  - ➤ Discovery of bradycardic, tachycardic or irregular rhythms

- Used to evaluate treatments:
  - ➤ Improvement in heart block
  - ➤ Successful cardioversion of **SVT**

84

Arrhythmias and Labor

Any rhythm disturbance has the potential to decrease fetal cardiac output.

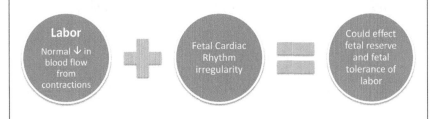

85

Comparison of Cardiac Characteristics

Factor	Fetus	Adult
Contractile mass	30%	60%
Calcium Transport	Altered	Fully functional
Cardiac Pressures	High on right side (atrium)	High on left side
Cardiac output (CO)	RV output + LV output	LV output
The fetus cannot alter stroke volume, therefore, fetal cardiac output is dependant on fetal heart RATE.		

86

Comparison of Cardiac Characteristics

Factor	Fetus	Adult
Contractile mass	30%	60%
Calcium Transport	Altered	Fully functional
Cardiac Pressures	High on right side (atrium)	High on left side
Cardiac output (CO)	RV output + LV output	LV output
The fetus cannot alter stroke volume, therefore, fetal cardiac output is dependant on fetal heart RATE.		

87

Adult ECG Pattern

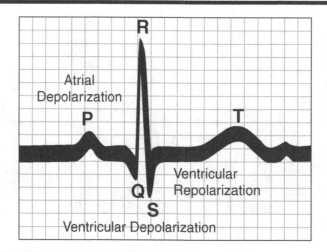

88

Cardiac Conduction System

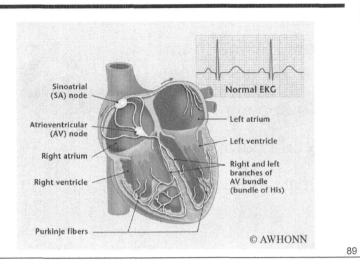

89

Cardiac Conduction System

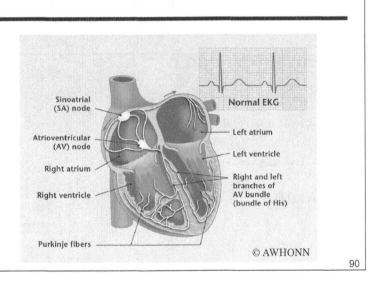

90

Potential Consequences of Fetal Arrhythmias

Potential continuum of consequences:

- No apparent effect

- Fetal hydrops

- Death

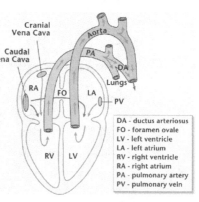

DA - ductus arteriosus
FO - foramen ovale
LV - left ventricle
LA - left atrium
RV - right ventricle
RA - right atrium
PA - pulmonary artery
PV - pulmonary vein

© AWHONN   91

Potential Consequences of Fetal Arrhythmias

Potential continuum of consequences:

- No apparent effect

- Fetal hydrops

- Death

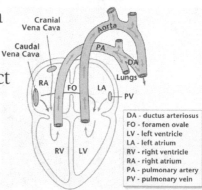

DA - ductus arteriosus
FO - foramen ovale
LV - left ventricle
LA - left atrium
RV - right ventricle
RA - right atrium
PA - pulmonary artery
PV - pulmonary vein

© AWHONN   92

Other Diagnostic Modalities

- Fetal echocardiography
- M-Mode echocardiogram

93

Other Diagnostic Modalities

- Pulsed Doppler echocardiogram
- Fetal magnetocardiography
- Tissue Doppler

94

Sinus Tachycardia

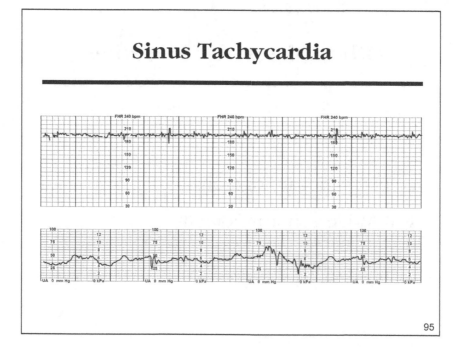

95

Sinus Tachycardia

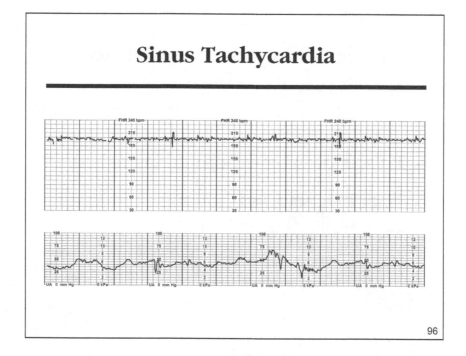

96

Sinus Bradycardia

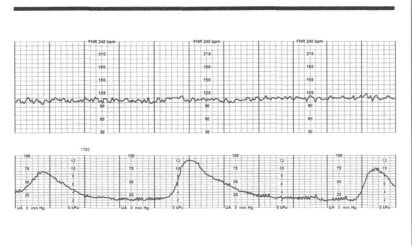

97

Sinus Bradycardia

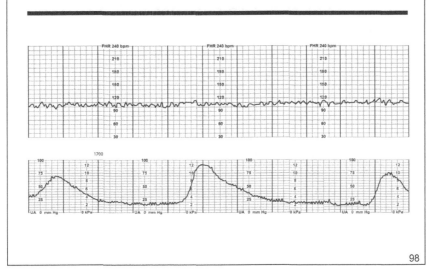

98

Atrioventricular (AV) Blocks

- Abnormal impulse conduction through the AV node

- Causes:
  - ➤ Cardiac structural damages
  - ➤ Maternal collagen vascular diseases
  - ➤ Fetal cytomegalovirus
  - ➤ Anti-phospholipid syndrome

99

Severity of AV Conduction Disorders

Severity:
- ➤ First degree *"Undetectable with EFM"*
  - Delayed impulse conduction (prolonged P-R interval)
- ➤ Second degree *"FHR may appear normal or have missed beats & spikes"*
  - Intermittent or occasional loss of conduction through the AV node
- ➤ Third degree *"Bradycardic FHR pattern"*:
  - Complete absence of impulse conduction from the SA node through the AV node
  - 50% of fetuses may have structural anomaly

100

Carmen

- G3P$_{22002}$, 30 weeks gestation
- 25 years old
- Transferred to MFM

101

Carmen: Studies

- Ultrasound—normal growth and anatomy, small amount fluid seen in pericardial sac; no others signs of hydrops
- M-Mode echocardiogram showed atrial rates in 130s and ventricular rates 60s–70s
- Confirming complete heart block
- Tests ordered—Lupus antibodies, anti-phospholipid antibody syndrome (APS) and TORCH titers
- Referral to pediatric cardiology

102

Carmen: 31 Weeks Gestation

- SSA/SSB antibodies positive
- BPP 8/8
- M-Mode echocardiogram:
  - ➢ Atrial rates 130s and ventricular rates 60s–70s
  - ➢ PR intervals normal
  - ➢ Second degree block with a 2:1 pattern *(two atrial contractions for every one ventricular contraction)*
- Treatment:
  - ➢ Dexamethasone 8 mg daily for 2 weeks, followed by 4 mg daily until delivery
- Follow up twice weekly

103

Carmen: Tracing 33 Weeks Gestation

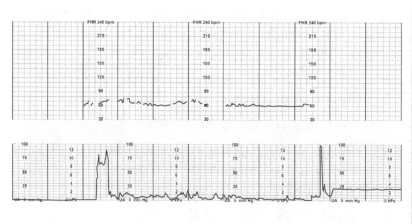

104

Carmen: Cardiologist Report @ 36 weeks

- Complete heart block:
  - ➤ Atrial rate regular 130 to 145 bpm
  - ➤ Ventricular rate of 60 to 70 bpm
- Right to left shunting of blood flow
- No ventricular septal defect
- Mild right ventricular enlargement with good biventricular contractility

105

Carmen: Cardiologist Report @ 36 Weeks

- Normal crossing of the great vessels
- Valves had normal diastolic inflow patterns with no regurgitation (tricuspid or mitral)
- Normal systolic flow across the semilunar valves
- No evidence of pleural, or pericardial effusions, ascites or skin edema

106

Carmen: 38 weeks
Day of Elective Cesarean Birth

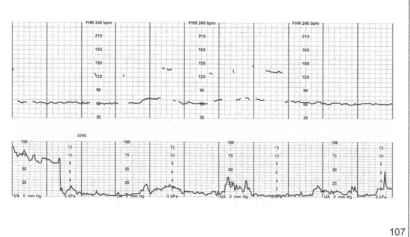

107

Carmen: Tracing Before Surgery

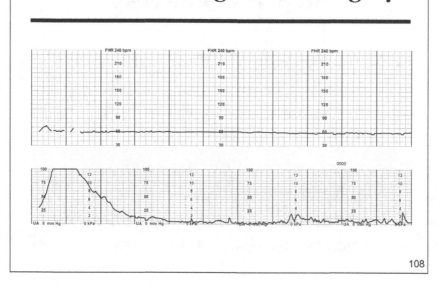

108

Carmen: Tracing Before Surgery

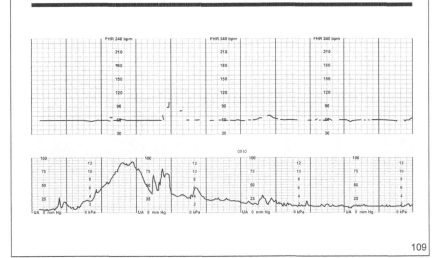

109

Delivery and Neonatal Outcome

- Infant delivers via Cesarean
- Apgar scores 8/9
- 5 minute pre-ductal O_2 sat 90% on room air
- T 98.4°F, HR 90 bpm, RR 45/min
- Discharged home after evaluation
- Stable heart rate in 70s; no pacing needed
- Cardiology follow up

110

Supraventricular Tachycardia (SVT)

- Non-sinus originated impulse:
  - ➤ Rates 210–320 bpm
    - Has been associated with Wolff–Parkinson White Syndrome
- Multiple electrical impulse pathways may occur in development of SVT
- Paroxysmal (occurring suddenly) or continuous

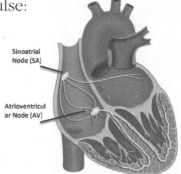

© AWHONN

111

SVT

- Increases workload of the fetal heart:
  - ➤ Increases cardiac oxygen demands
  - ➤ Decreases cardiac output
  - ➤ Increased hemolysis of RBCs' that reduce oxygen delivery
  - ➤ All may lead to heart failure

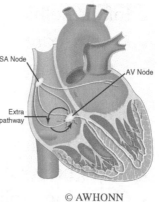

© AWHONN

112

Cardiac arrhythmia

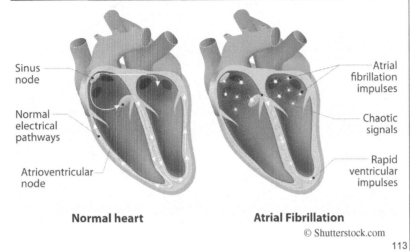

Sinus node

Normal electrical pathways

Atrioventricular node

Atrial fibrillation impulses

Chaotic signals

Rapid ventricular impulses

Normal heart

Atrial Fibrillation

© Shutterstock.com

113

SVT vs. Atrial Flutter

SVT:
- Due to reentry impulses around a circular pathway involving the AV node
- Has a 1:1 P:QRS ratio

Atrial flutter:
Due to reentry impulses around a circular pathway within atrium; does not involve AV node Atrial flutter is usually 2:1 but can have 3:1, 4:1, and variable P:QRS ratio

114

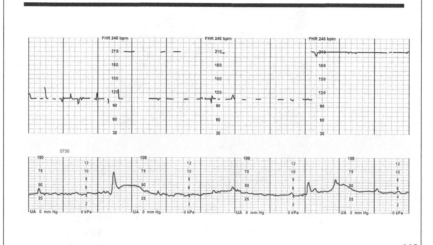

SVT vs. Atrial Flutter

115

Lilly

- 25 years old

- G3P$_{22002}$

- 30 weeks gestation

- Seen in rural community beginning @ 12 weeks gestation

116

Lilly

- Past medical history
  - ➤ + Asthma—prn use of Albuterol
- Social history:
  - ➤ Lives with the father of baby
  - ➤ Nonsmoker, denies drugs use, stopped drinking alcohol at 4 weeks gestation

117

Lilly

- Obstetrical history:
  - ➤ 2 spontaneous term vaginal deliveries
  - ➤ Chlamydia + during this pregnancy (treated to cure for both patient and partner)
- Transferred to tertiary care center at 30 weeks gestation for MFM evaluation and treatment of fetal tachycardia

118

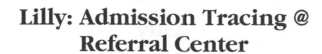

Lilly: Admission Tracing @ Referral Center

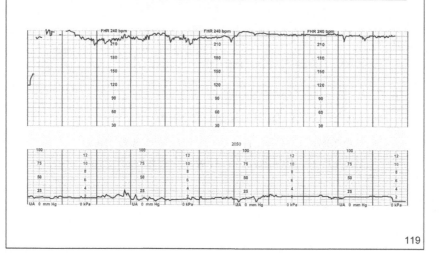

119

Lilly: On Day Four of Therapy

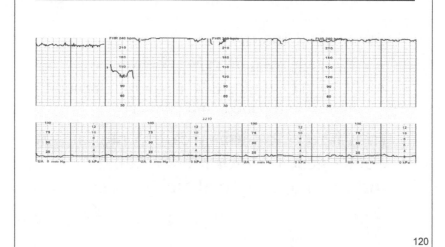

120

Lilly: On Day Nine of Therapy

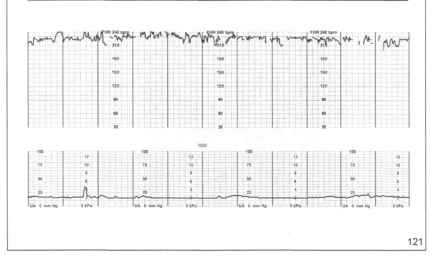

121

Lilly: On Day 15 of Therapy

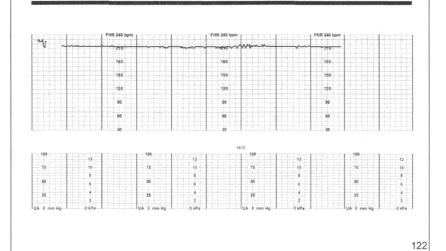

122

Lilly: Fetal Ultrasound On Delivery Day

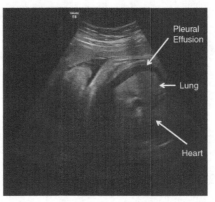

Pleural
Effusion

Lung

Heart

Used with permission from Cindy Cochrane

123

Neonatal Outcome

- Male infant born by Cesarean at 32.6 weeks gestation
- Apgar scores 8/9
- Delayed cord clamping for 60 seconds
- 2639 g (5 lbs. 13.1 oz.)
- Placed on CPAP
- Temp 98.4°F, HR 183 bpm, RR 46/min
- Admit to cardiac NICU

124

Premature Atrial Contractions and Premature Ventricular

	Premature Atrial Contractions (PAC)	Premature Ventricular Contractions (PVC)
Cardiac physiology bigeminy and trigeminy can occur with both PAC and PVC	• Conducted: premature P wave following by a normal QRS complex • Non-conducted: PAC is too premature to move through the AV node but causes a premature depolarization followed by a compensatory pause.	• An ectopic ventricular focus producing a ventricular contraction independent of the SA node. • May be followed by a compensatory pause when the ventricles cannot respond to stimuli form the SA node. Respiratory depression
Causes	Redundancy or aneurysm of the flap covering the foraman ovale, maternal caffeine, nicotine, alcohol use or hyperthyroidism	Fetal hydrops, cardiomyopathies, myocarditis, digitalis toxicity, maternal use of caffeine, nicotine, alcohol or cocaine. Rare hypokalemia from maternal hyperemesis.
Treatment the same for both	Avoid maternal caffeine, nicotine, alcohol, sympathomimetic medications and illicit drugs. * Both may resolve spontaneously	

125

Premature Atrial Contractions and Premature Ventricular

	Premature Atrial Contractions (PAC)	Premature Ventricular Contractions (PVC)
Cardiac physiology bigeminy and trigeminy can occur with both PAC and PVC	• Conducted: premature P wave following by a normal QRS complex • Non-conducted: PAC is too premature to move through the AV node but causes a premature depolarization followed by a compensatory pause.	• An ectopic ventricular focus producing a ventricular contraction independent of the SA node. • May be followed by a compensatory pause when the ventricles cannot respond to stimuli form the SA node. Respiratory depression
Causes	Redundancy or aneurysm of the flap covering the foraman ovale, maternal caffeine, nicotine, alcohol use or hyperthyroidism	Fetal hydrops, cardiomyopathies, myocarditis, digitalis toxicity, maternal use of caffeine, nicotine, alcohol or cocaine. Rare hypokalemia from maternal hyperemesis.
Treatment the same for both	Avoid maternal caffeine, nicotine, alcohol, sympathomimetic medications and illicit drugs. * Both may resolve spontaneously	

126

Premature Atrial Contractions and Premature Ventricular Contractions

EFM Findings:

- Both PAC and PVC's are seen on EFM as vertical spikes.

- The upward spike is the premature beat and the downward spike is the compensatory pause.

- The baseline FHR will be seen intermittently between these upward and downward strokes.

- You cannot differentiate between PAC's or PVC's with EFM.

127

Antonia

- 33 years old
- G2 P$_{10101}$
- 38 weeks gestation
- Admitted:
  - SROM and irregular contractions
  - Cervix 2 cm/80%/0 station
  - EFW 7 lbs.
- Medical history
  - Tonsillectomy age 6 years

128

Antonia

- Obstetrical history:
  - Cesarean delivery @ 36 weeks due to breech presentation
- Current pregnancy:
  - Adequate prenatal visits:
    - Denies smoking, alcohol, or substance abuse
    - Prenatal labs WNL except GBS+
- Plan TOLAC:
  - PCN for GBS prophylaxis
  - Epidural as desired when in active labor

129

Antonia: Admission Tracing

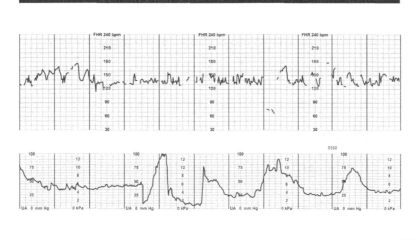

130

Antonia: 0634

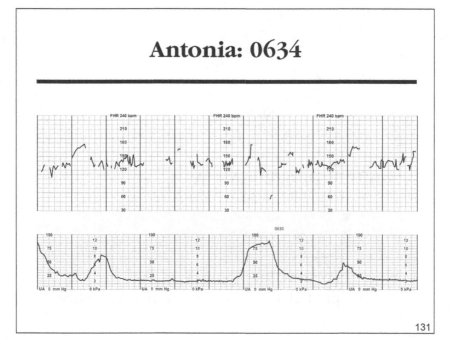

131

Clinical Responsibilities

- Establish FHR baseline and other characteristics if possible

- Document audible changes, irregularities

- Notify the primary providers neonatologists/pediatrician/NNP

132

Antonia

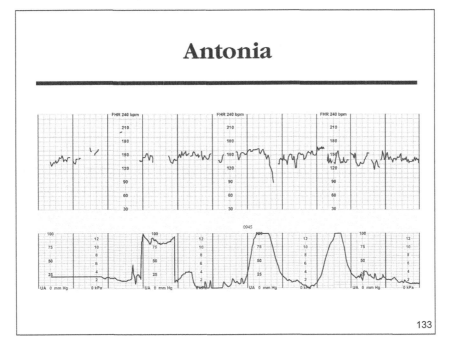

133

Antonia: After Epidural

134

Antonia

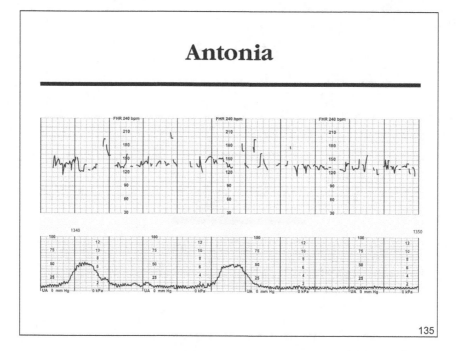

135

Antonia

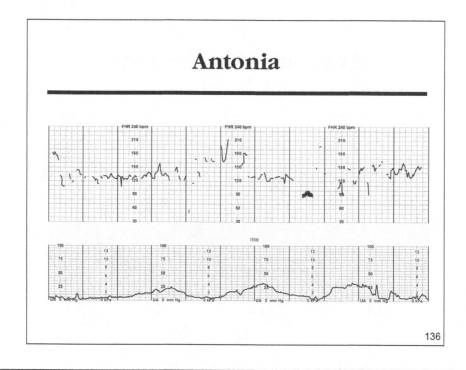

136

Antonia: With FSE

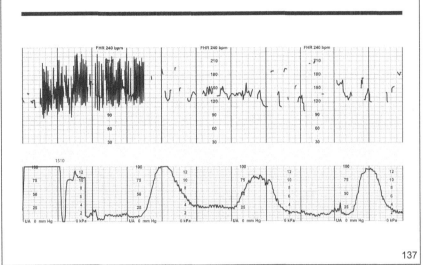

137

Antonia

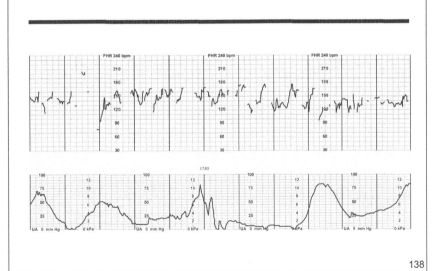

138

Antonia

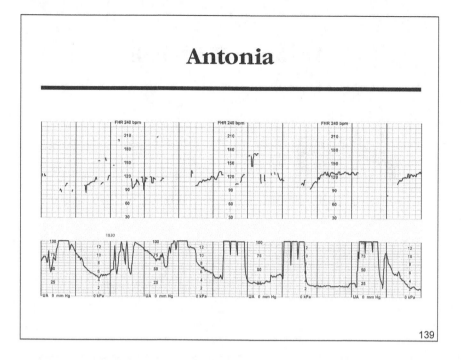

139

Antonia: 1854

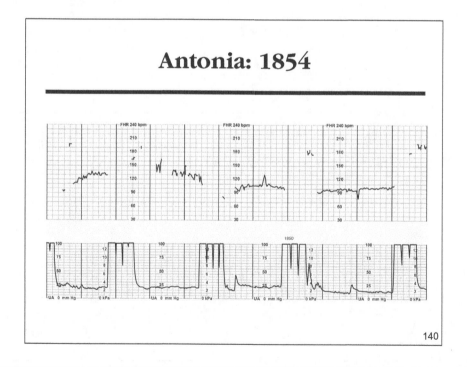

140

Outcomes

- Delivery @ 1859:
  - Successful VBAC
  - Bilateral labial tears repaired
  - QBL 250 ml
- Male Infant
  - 7lbs 9oz, 19.5"
- Apgar scores 8 and 9:
  - Infant vigorous
  - Nuchal cord X1

- Infant day 2 of life:
  - 12 lead EKG showed multiple PVCs
  - Infant referred to cardiology
    - Repeat EKG in 2 weeks
- Both mother and infant discharged on postpartum day 2

141

Arrhythmia Conclusion

- Incidence is rare
- Effects on fetal cardiac output and fetal oxygenation
- Outcomes variable
- Medical management
- Nursing management
- EFM and fetal arrhythmias

142

Complex Case Scenarios

143

Umbilical Cord Blood Interpretation Review

Acidosis	pH	pCO₂	Base Deficit	Base Excess
Respiratory	Low pH (< 7.10)	High pCO₂ (> 60)	Normal (< 12)	Normal (> −12)
Metabolic	Low pH (< 7.10)	Normal pCO₂ (< 60)	High (≥ 12)	Low (≤ − 12)
Mixed	Low pH (< 7.10)	High pCO₂ (> 60)	High (≥ 12)	Low (≤ − 12)

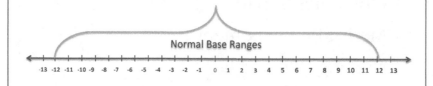

Normal Base Ranges

-13 -12 -11 -10 -9 -8 -7 -6 -5 -4 -3 -2 -1 0 1 2 3 4 5 6 7 8 9 10 11 12 13

144

Brittany

- G_1P_0
- 37 3/7 weeks gestation
- Family history:
  - Paternal: bipolar, diabetes
  - Maternal: alcoholism

145

Brittany

- Medical history:
  - History of depression
  - Penicillin allergy
- Social history:
  - Married
  - Denies tobacco, alcohol, or drug uses

146

Brittany: Admission Tracing

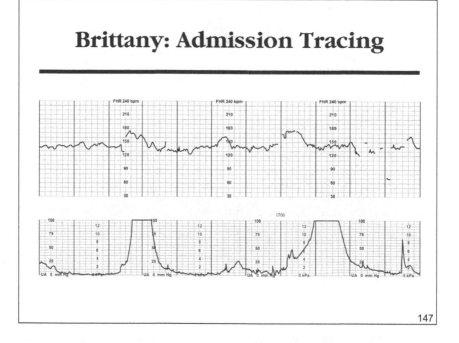

147

Brittany: Admission Tracing

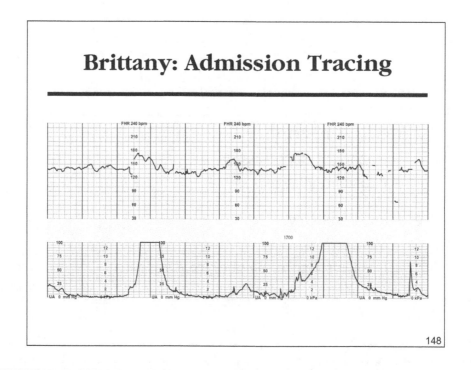

148

Brittany: 2248

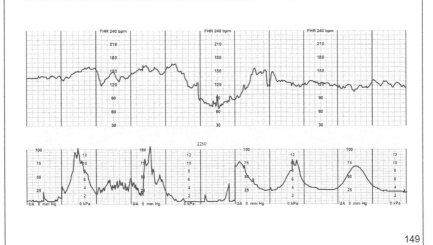

149

Brittany

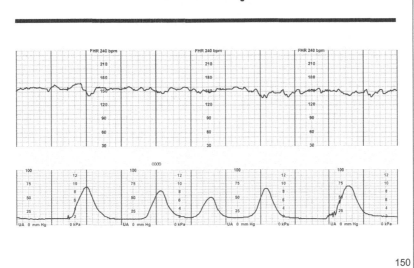

150

Brittany

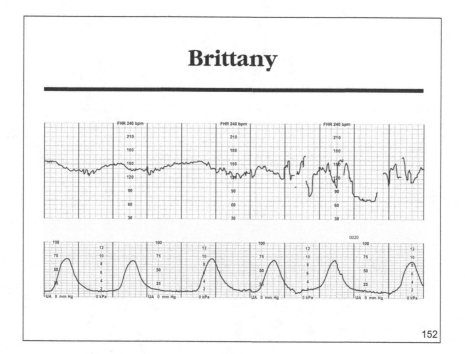

151

Brittany

152

Brittany

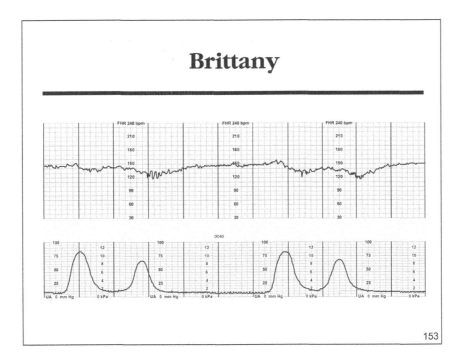

153

Brittany: 0100

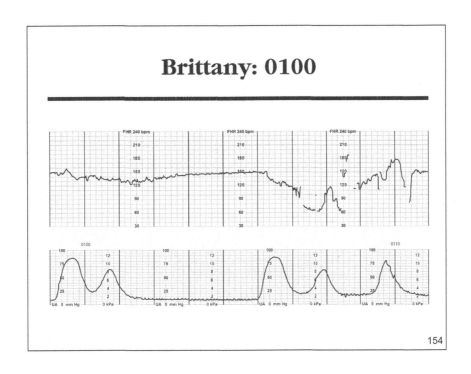

154

Brittany: 0100

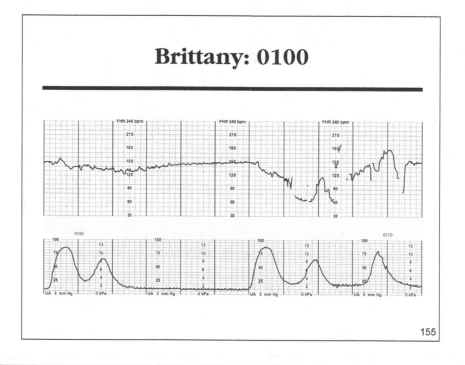

155

Brittany

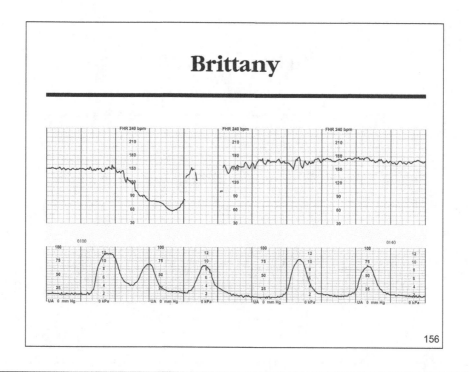

156

Brittany

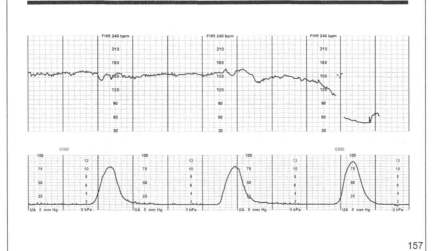

157

Brittany: Newborn Outcome

- Male infant
- Cord around body
- Apgar scores 7 and 8
- Arterial cord gases:
  - ➢ pH 6.95
  - ➢ pCO2 115
  - ➢ HCO3 24.4
  - ➢ Base excess –11

- 6 lbs. 7.7 oz.
- To NICU to transition then to general nursery
  - ➢ Home on day 4

158

Brittany: Outcome

- Tolerated surgical delivery
- QBL 700 ml
- Transferred intubated to ICU
- Extubated after 8 hours
- Transferred to mother/baby unit

- Mild anoxic brain injury:
  - Short-term memory loss
  - Normal EEG and brain CT scans
  - 2 normal echocardiograms
- Discharged on day 4
- Short-term memory loss resolved

159

Brittany: Outcome

- Tolerated surgical delivery
- QBL 700 ml
- Transferred intubated to ICU
- Extubated after 8 hours
- Transferred to mother/baby unit

- Mild anoxic brain injury:
  - Short-term memory loss
  - Normal EEG and brain CT scans
  - 2 normal echocardiograms
- Discharged on day 4
- Short-term memory loss resolved

160

Cardiac Arrest in Pregnancy

- Incidence: 1:12,000

161

Cardiac Arrest in Pregnancy

- Basic and advanced cardiac life support:
  - ➤ Early ventilatory support
  - ➤ Left uterine displacement

162

Cardiac Arrest in Pregnancy

- No fetal assessment
- Perimortem cesarean delivery
- Multidisciplinary team response

163

Cardiac Arrest in Pregnancy

- Multiple etiologies

164

Tatiana

- 20 years old
- G2 P$_{10101}$
- 37 3/7 weeks' gestation
- Weight 197 lbs., height 5'4"
- Family history unremarkable

165

Tatiana

Medical and obstetrical history:
- Spontaneous vaginal delivery 3 years ago @ 36 weeks gestation; complicated with preeclampsia
- States, "I had baby blues after my first baby was born"
- Previous smoker one pack per day; quit with pregnancy

166

Tatiana: Admission Data

- Irregular contractions and spontaneous rupture of membranes

- Vital signs
  - BP 122/67, P 93 bpm, R 20/min, T 98.4°F

167

Tatiana: Admission Data

- Physical exam:
  - Cervix: soft, midline, 3 cm, 60%, −2 station, cephalic presentation
  - Nitrazine positive
  - Moderate amount clear fluid noted

168

Tatiana: 0445 Tracing

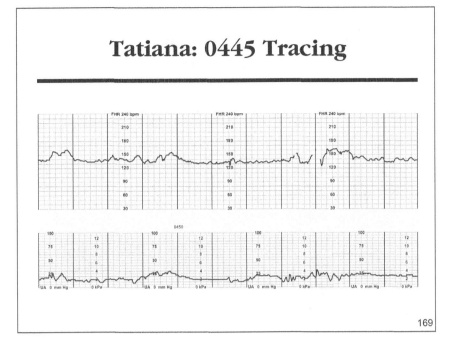

Tatiana: 0800

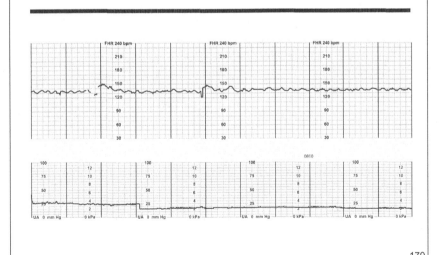

Sinusoidal vs Sinusoidal-Appearing

	Etiologies	Characteristics	Treatment
Sinusoidal Fetal Heart Pattern	Severe fetal anemia due to Rh isoimmunization Massive fetomaternal hemorrhage Twin to twin transfusion syndrome Ruptured vasa previa Fetal intracranial hemorrhage Fetal hypoxia or asphyxia Fetal infection Fetal cardiac anomalies Gastroschisis	• Visually apparent, undulating, smooth sine wave-like pattern in the FHR baseline with a cycle frequency of 3–5 per minute that persists for at least 20 minutes • No accelerations and no FHR responses to uterine contractions, fetal movement, or stimulation	Requires immediate attention
Sinusoidal-Appearing Fetal Heart Pattern	Maternal administration of some opioids (especially butorphanol and fentanyl) Fetal sleep cycles Fetal thumb sucking Rhythmic movements of the fetal mouth.	Usually undulating FHR pattern is of short duration and is both preceded and followed by an FHR with normal characteristics	No treatment is indicated for sinusoidal-appearing patterns when history of maternal opioid administration is clearly related to the following tracing.

* The term pseudosinusoidal is not an NICHD approved terminology

171

Tatiana: 1230

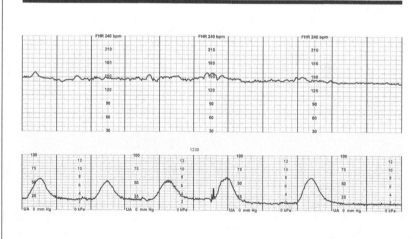

172

Tatiana: 1615

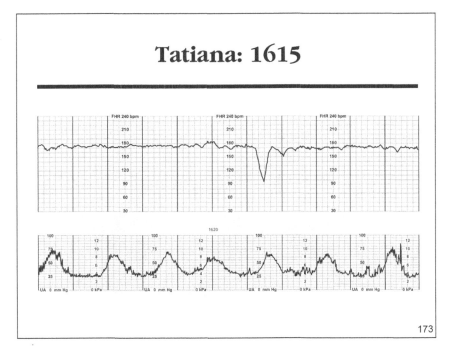

173

Tatiana: 1615

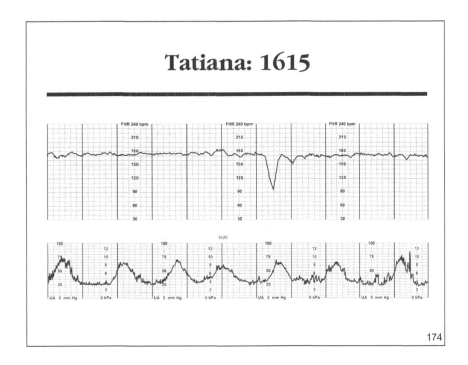

174

Tatiana: 1700

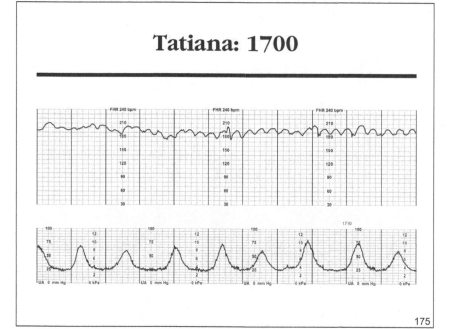

175

Fever

- Epidural analgesia is the most common cause of increased maternal temperature

- There is evidence that pyrexia (no matter the cause) during labor increases risk of neonatal encephalopathy

176

Fever

- Epidural analgesia is the most common cause of increased maternal temperature

- There is evidence that pyrexia (no matter the cause) during labor increases risk of neonatal encephalopathy

177

Tatiana: 1735

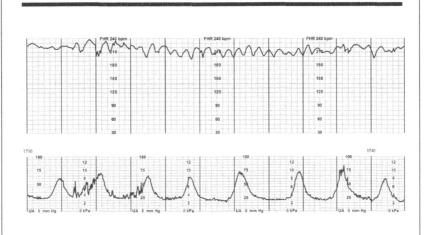

178

Tatiana: 1800

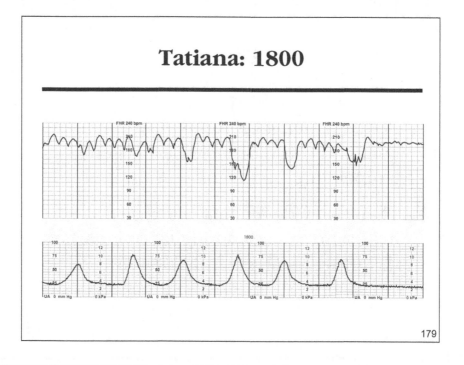

179

Tatiana: 1910

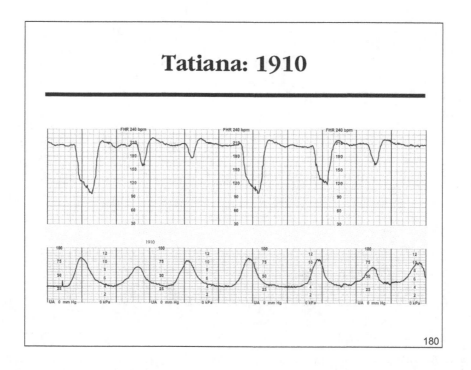

180

Tatiana

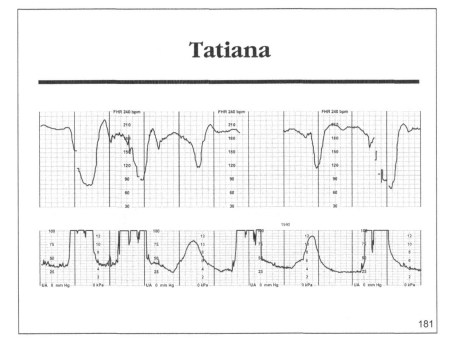

181

Tatiana: 1955

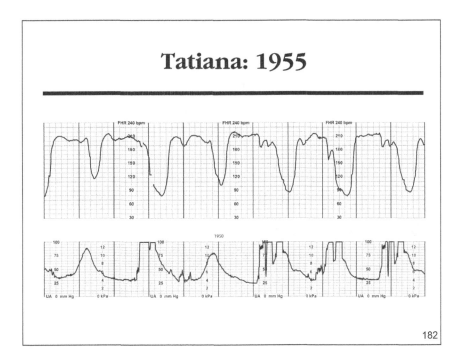

182

Tatiana: Outcomes

- Spontaneous vaginal delivery
- Male 8 lbs. 6 oz.
- Apgar scores 6 and 8 (normal cord gases):
  - ➢ Nuchal cord ×1, easily reduced
  - ➢ Meconium stained fluid at delivery
  - ➢ Grunting @ 5 minutes of age
- Transferred to NICU:
  - ➢ Bubble CPAP for 24 hours
  - ➢ IV antibiotic for 48 hours until blood cultures determined negative
- Discharged 5 days of life

183

Heather

- 38 years old
- G_3P_{2002}
- 38 weeks gestation
- Family history:
  - ➢ Paternal: HTN, heart disease
  - ➢ Maternal: breast cancer

184

Heather

Medical and obstetrical history:

- ➤ No surgeries or chronic illness
- ➤ Two previous term, vaginal deliveries 13 and 8 years ago
  - Hematoma with first delivery and no complications with second birth

- Social history:
  - ➤ Married, no smoking, alcohol or drugs

185

Heather: Admission Data

- Spontaneous contractions:
  - ➤ Intact membranes; hydramnios
  - ➤ Cervix: 2 cm, 50%, −2 station and breech presentation
  - ➤ EFW 8 lbs.
  - ➤ Vital signs:
    - Temp 98.2°F, pulse 88 bpm, RR 18/min, BP 119/66
    - Pain score 1/10
  - ➤ Height 5'4" weight 185 lbs.

186

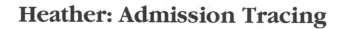

Heather: Admission Tracing

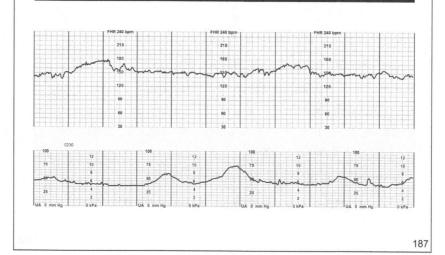

187

External Cephalic Version

- Attempted before labor ≥ 37 weeks

- Ultrasound confirms presentation

- Informed consent obtained for procedure and use of tocolytics

- NST to established fetal status and contraction pattern

188

External Cephalic Version

- In setting where emergent Cesarean can be performed

- Contraindicated if vaginal delivery not appropriate

189

Heather: Tracing After Version

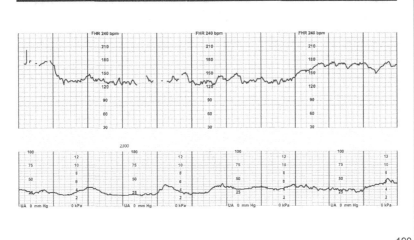

190

Heather: 0300

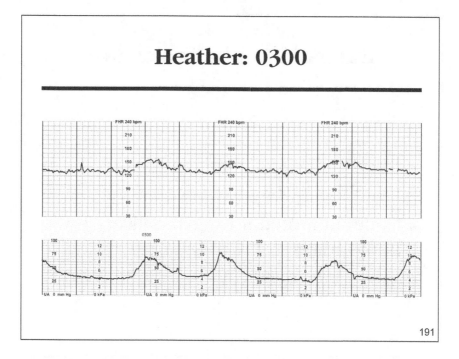

191

Heather: 0645

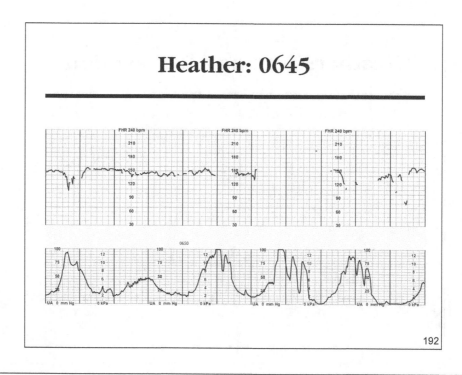

192

Heather: 0820

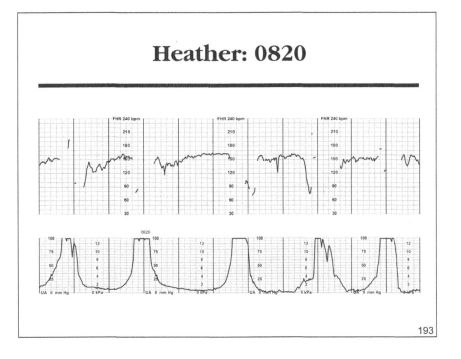

193

Heather: 0840

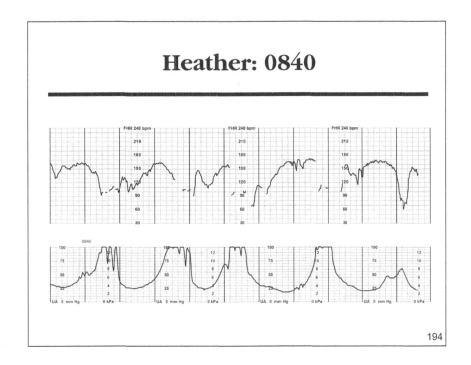

194

Heather: 0900

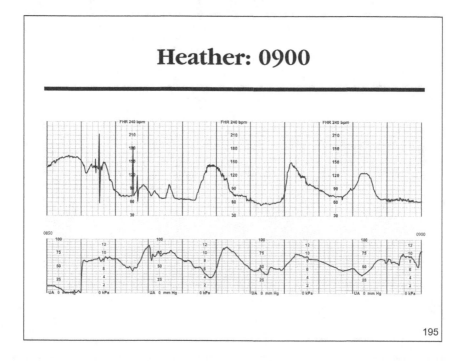

Heather: Prior to Transfer to OR

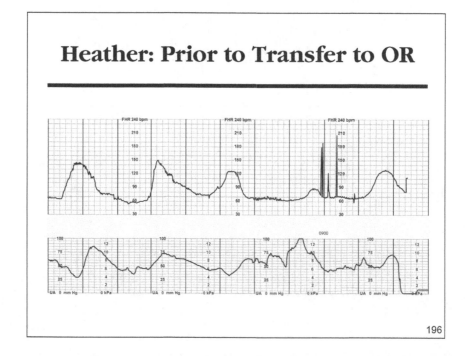

Heather: Outcomes

- Cesarean birth @ 0918

- Female infant, 8 lbs. 2.5 oz.

- Apgar scores 2/6/8

- Large posterior uterine rupture noted in midline of uterus

- QBL 1500 ml

197

Heather: Outcomes

Umbilical arterial cord gases

	Arterial	Venous
pH	6.8	6.9
pCO_2	100	82.4
pO_2	20	20
HCO_3	?	17.9
BE	?	−14

198

Uterine Rupture

- Fetal heart rate changes:
  - ➤ Bradycardia
  - ➤ Bradycardia preceded by variable or late decelerations
- Abdominal pain with/without hemodynamic changes:
  - ➤ Hypotension, tachycardia, increasing abdominal girth
  - ➤ Hemoperitoneum may cause chest pain due to irritation of diaphragm
- Uterine tenderness, cessation of contractions, change in uterine shape
- Vaginal bleeding or hematuria
- Loss of fetal station

199

Uterine Rupture Risk Factors

- Previous cesarean deliveries
- Trauma
- Factors in perinatal history
- Fetal factors

200

Shondra

- 21 years old

- G_2P_{10101}

- Family history:
  - ➤ Maternal-diabetic
  - ➤ Paternal-hypertension

201

Shondra

- Obstetrical history:
  - ➤ Previous vaginal delivery, medical induction @ 32 weeks followed by eclamptic seizure

- Social history:
  - ➤ Married, denies smoking, alcohol or drug use
  - ➤ 2-year-old child developmentally delayed

202

Shondra Current Pregnancy

- Prenatal lab values
- Medications

203

Shondra: Triage Visit

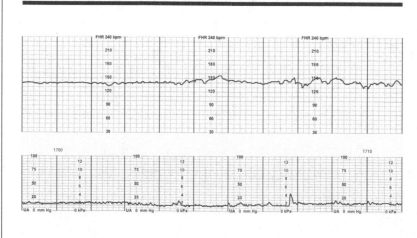

204

Shondra: Serial BP's and Labs

Time	BP	Position
1623	142/91	Low Fowlers
1635	134/89	
1645	164/88	
1656	132/80	
1705	135/87	
Lab test	**Results**	
Urine protein	+1	
Nitrite, blood, Ketones, glucose	Trace	
Leukocyte estrace	Trace	

205

Shondra: Second OB Triage Visit

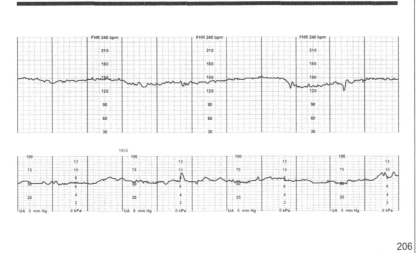

206

Shondra

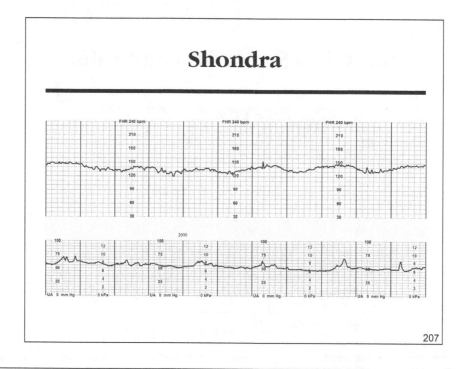

207

Shondra

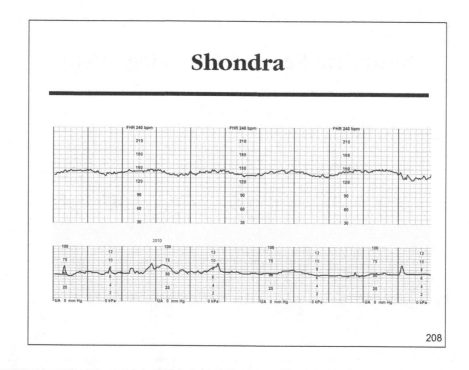

208

Shondra

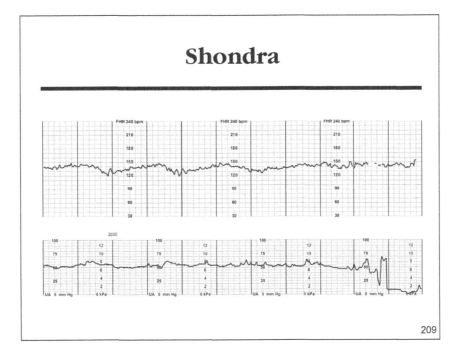

Shondra

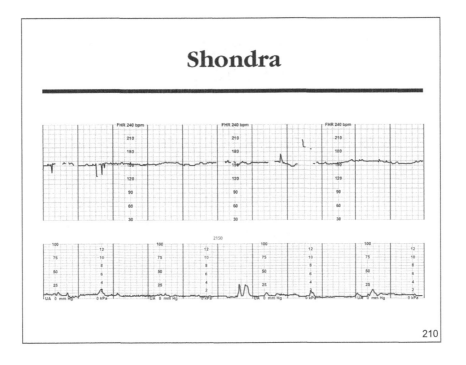

Shondra

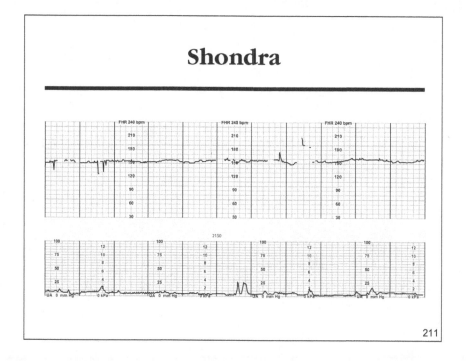

211

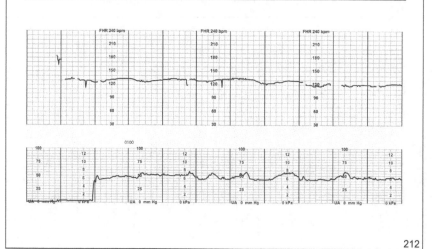

Shondra: Two Hours After Discharge

212

Shondra

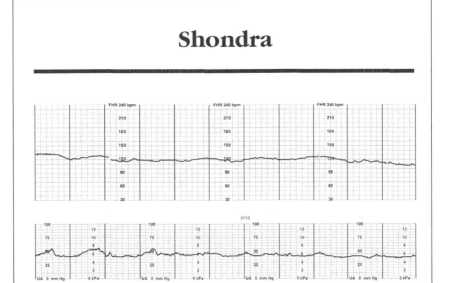

213

Shondra

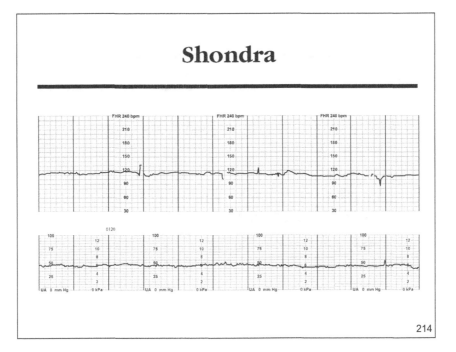

214

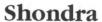

Shondra

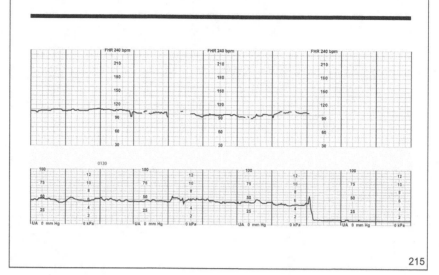

215

Shondra: Outcomes

- 0143 auscultated FHR in OR 93 bpm after removal of EFM
- 0145 Cesarean delivery with general anesthesia
- Male infant, 3 lbs. 7oz; poor tone and pale color
  - ➤ Apgar 0/2/2 @ 1/5/10 minutes
- Bloody amniotic fluid
- 75% placental abruption:
  - ➤ Couvelaire uterus
  - ➤ QBL 1000 ml

216

Shondra Umbilical Cord Gases

	Venous	Arterial
pH	6.876	6.782
pCO_2	85.5	100
PO_2	24	20
HCO_3	16	Unable to calculate
Base excess	−17	Unable to calculate

217

Abruptio Placenta

Risk factors:
— Prior abruption
— Preeclampsia
— Chronic hypertension
— Chorioamnionitis
— Premature rupture

Risk factors:
— Low birth weight
— Hydramnios
— Cigarette smoking
— Thrombophilias
— Cocaine use
  of membranes
— Uterine leiomyoma
— Trauma

218

Abruptio Placenta

Clinical findings:
— Sudden-onset of abdominal pain
— Vaginal bleeding
— Uterine tenderness
— Back pain
— FHR characteristics of interrupted oxygenation
— Frequent uterine contractions
— Persistent uterine hypertonus

219

Charlotte

- 16 years old
- G1P0
- Family history:
  ➤ Charlotte was adopted
- Medical and obstetrical history:
  ➤ Uses inhaler prn for asthma
  ➤ Prenatal care began at 28 weeks gestation
- Social history:
  ➤ Lived with friends until moved back home with parents
  ➤ Completed 10th grade

220

Charlotte

Prenatal laboratory studies:

- HPV positive

- Chlamydia positive

- GBS +

- Abnormal pap smear

- Rubella non-immune

221

Charlotte

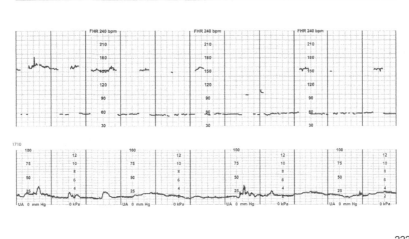

222

Charlotte

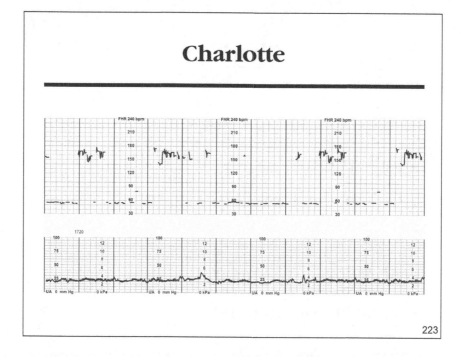

223

Charlotte: Admission

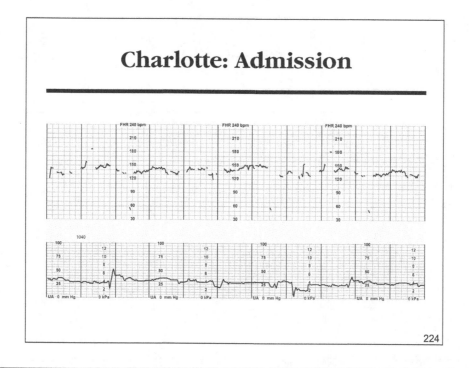

224

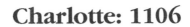

Charlotte: 1106

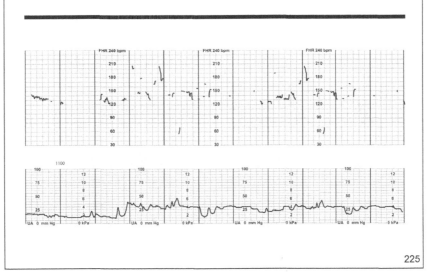

225

Charlotte

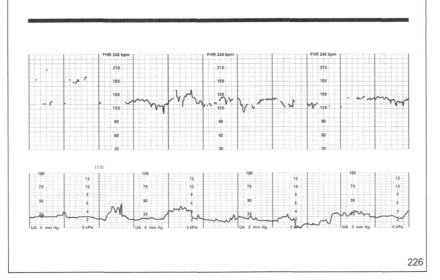

226

Charlotte

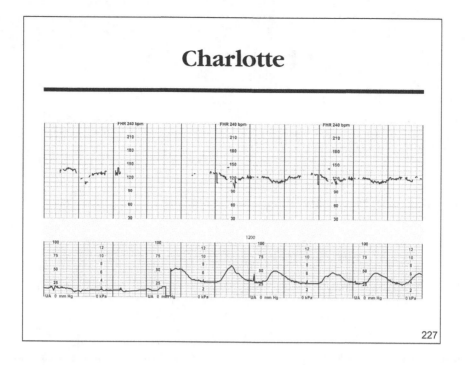

227

Charlotte

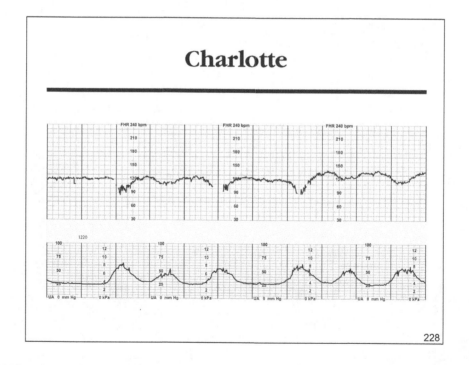

228

Charlotte

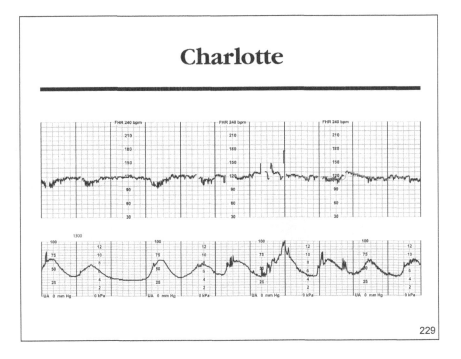

229

Charlotte

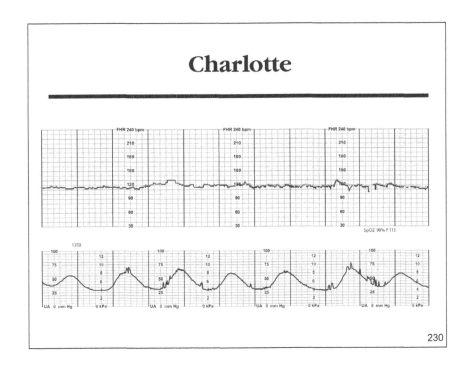

230

Charlotte

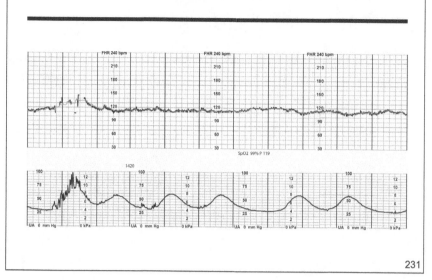

231

Charlotte: Delivery

- Vaginal delivery
  - ➤ Male stillborn

- Placenta cultures to lab:
  - ➤ Aerobic and anaerobic fetal and maternal sides
  - ➤ Tissue culture of placenta for Listeria

232

Charlotte: Postpartum

- Elevated WBC
- Normal test results for:
  - Cardiolipin antibody (IgG and IgM)
  - Creatinine
  - Urine drug screen
  - HSV I and II (IgM and IgG)
  - CMV (IgM and IgG)
  - Parvovirus B19 antibody (IgM and IgG)
  - Rubella (IgM and IgG)
  - Toxoplasma antibody (IgM and IgG):
    - ✓ N. Gonorrhoeae
    - ✓ Chlamydia trachomatis

233

Opportunities

- Difficulty in assessment of fetal heart rate:
  - Assess maternal heart rate with every application of EFM
    - Be cautious when MHR is in range of a normal FHR
      - ✓ Utilize EFM capabilities of tracing MHR when available
  - Use methods to troubleshoot ultrasound transducer
  - Ask for provider assistance with ultrasound
  - In the presence of fetal demise, the maternal ECG signal will be picked up by the fetal spiral electrode

234

Summary

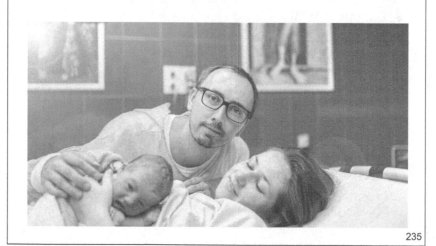

235

Teamwork, Communication and Documentation

236

Teamwork

- Requires commitment to quality and best possible outcomes

- Disallows disruptive behaviors

237

Teamwork

- TeamSTEPPS™:
  - ➤ Leadership
  - ➤ Situation monitoring
  - ➤ Mutual support

238

Teamwork

➤ Communication:
- Call-out
- Check-back (closing the loop)

239

Teamwork

- Sharing the plan
  - ➤ Brief

- Monitoring and modifying the plan
  - ➤ Huddle

- Reviewing the team's performance
  - ➤ Debrief

240

Communication

- Exchange of information

- May be verbal, written, electronic

- Essential in perinatal teamwork:
  - ➢ Supports delivery of safe care
  - ➢ Quality influences outcomes

241

Communication

- Competency in communication skills and clinical skills equally important

- Key component of any safety program

- Clinicians have the obligation to speak up

242

Structured Communication

- Formats often used:
  - ➢ SBAR
  - ➢ SBAR-R
  - ➢ SBAR-R-R

243

Structured Communication

➢ SBAR for listening:
  - Set aside assumptions
  - Be attentive
  - Ask questions
  - Reflect

244

Structured Communication

- Critical language:
  - ➤ Neutral phrase
  - ➤ Signals the team
  - ➤ May be used in presence of the patient
- CUS:
  - ➤ I am concerned
  - ➤ I am uncomfortable
  - ➤ This is a safety issue

245

Electronic Fetal Monitoring Communication

- NICHD terminology endorsed by professional associations

- FHR assessments communicated using NICHD terminology

- Communication and safety promoted through interdisciplinary education

246

Electronic Fetal Monitoring Communication

- Nurses, physicians and midwives learning together enhances collaboration:
  - ➤ Decreases frequency of disagreement
  - ➤ Increases opportunity for interaction
  - ➤ Increases understanding of one another's perspectives

247

Communication with Patients

- Inquire about woman's wishes
- Be respectful for the dignity of the woman and family
- Involve interpreters/translators/cultural preferences
- Include the woman in decisions when possible

248

Fetal Monitoring Decisions

- Inquire about preferences for monitoring

- Begin with the least invasive method of monitoring

- Prepare the woman for changes in monitoring that may occur during labor

249

Patient Handoffs

- During transfer of patient from one care provider to another

- Intended to promote continuity and efficiency

- Standardization supports patient safety and reduces communication breakdowns

250

Strategies for Promoting Safe Handoffs

- Utilize face-to-face communication
- Assess the patient together
- Limit interruptions
- Delay transfer if there are concerns
- Remain present during emergencies until there is assurance all critical information has been transferred and received

251

Conflict Management

- Focus on commitment to the woman
- Support mutual emphasis on achieving optimal outcomes
- Keep in mind that professionalism includes mutual respect and trust

252

Conflict Management

- Difficult conversations—consider timing and context
- Choose an appropriate location
- Attend to body language and verbal cues
- Avoid defensiveness

253

Conflict Management

- Clarify the differing points of view
- Listen attentively
- Avoid interruptions
- Ask clarifying questions
- Summarize understanding of the other person's communication

254

Chain of Resolution

- Clinicians should know organizational policies

- Initial link is conversation between the nurse and physician

- Move to the next step if solution is not achieved

255

Chain of Resolution

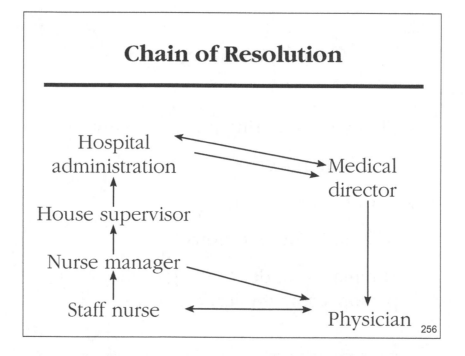

256

Chain of Resolution

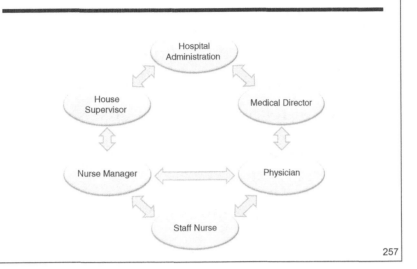

257

Documentation

- Documentation:
    - Communicates patient's status
    - Conveys information to the health-care team
    - Should be accurate, timely
    - Should include patient's responses to care provided

258

Documentation

- Accuracy and thoroughness decrease liability

- Medical record role in defense

- Medical record role in documenting adverse events

  But . . . care comes first in emergencies

259

Documentation

- Should be systematic
- Include assessment of mother and fetus
- Ongoing:
  - ➤ Fetal information
  - ➤ Uterine activity
  - ➤ Interventions
  - ➤ Evaluation of responses

260

Documentation

- Should include:
  - ➢ Communication with woman and her support persons
  - ➢ Communication with providers
  - ➢ Communication within the chain of resolution process

261

Intermittent Auscultation

Table 1: Recommendations for Assessment and Documentation of Fetal Status during Labor When Using Intermittent Auscultation[a]

	Latent phase (< 4 cm)	Latent phase (4–5 cm)	Active phase (> 6 cm)	Second stage (passive fetal descent)	Second stage (active pushing)
Low-risk, without oxytocin	At least hourly	Every 15–30 minutes	Every 15–30 minutes	Every 15 minutes	Every 5–15 minutes

262

Fetal Assessments During Labor Using Electronic Fetal Monitoring

Low-risk, without oxytocin	At least hourly during latent phase (< 4 cm.)	Every 30 minutes during latent phase (4–5 cm)	Every 30 minutes during active phase (≥ 6 cm)	Every 15minutes during second stage (passive fetal descent)	Every 15 minutes during second stage (active pushing)
With oxytocin or risk factors	Every 15 minutes with oxytocin; every 30 minutes without during latent phase (< 4 cm)	Every 15 minutes during latent phase (4–5 cm)	Every 15 minutes during active phase (≥ 6 cm)	Every 15 minutes during second stage (passive fetal descent)	Every 5 minutes during second stage (active pushing)

263

Documentation of FHR Characteristics

AUSCULTATION	ELECTRONIC MONITORING
Rate	Rate
Rhythm	Variability
Increases and Decreases	Periodic and Episodic Changes
	Pattern Evolution
Associated clinical findings	
Communications	

264

Documenting Uterine Activity

Palpation	Tocodynamometer	Intrauterine Pressure Catheter
Frequency In minutes from beginning of one contraction to the beginning of the next		
Duration In seconds: average length of contractions		
Soft or firm	Resting Tone By palpation: soft, firm	mmHg <u>and</u> palpation
Mild, moderate, strong	Intensity Mild, moderate, strong	mmHg <u>and</u> palpation
DescriptiveDegree of associated pain and maternal coping *Normal uterine activity or Tachysystole*		

265

Electronic Documentation

- Format facilitates accessibility
- Federal legislation intended to improve care by use of health information technology
- Incentives provided for organizations that report required data

266

Electronic Documentation

- Advantages:
  - ➤ Rapid access
  - ➤ Improved accuracy and quality
  - ➤ Decreases in medical errors
  - ➤ Improved collection of coding and billing processes
  - ➤ Negates need for paper filing and record retention

267

Electronic Documentation

- Challenges:
  - ➤ Considerable financial investment
  - ➤ Cost and time required for clinician education
  - ➤ Require maintenance, upgrades and interfaces
  - ➤ "Downtime" processes necessary when unavailable

268

Flow Sheets and Narrative Notes

- Flow sheets:
  - ➤ Design should prompt notations
  - ➤ Should be consistent with unit guidelines
  - ➤ Reflect same content as paper flow sheets

- Narrative notes:
  - ➤ Capture what is not in flow sheet

- Summary documentation

269

Checklists

- Used to promote safety and reduce complications

- Multiple forms:
  - ➤ Surgical records
  - ➤ Induction readiness
  - ➤ Time out documentation
  - ➤ Procedural cues

270

Audits of Medical Records

- Promote accurate and timely documentation

- Support evaluation of adherence to documentation guidelines

- Provide valuable insight into tracing interpretation and patient care

271

Informed Consent

- Informed consent:
  - ➢ Form of communication
  - ➢ Represents discussion between medical care provider and patient
  - ➢ Not merely a form
  - ➢ Emergencies may limit achievement
  - ➢ Not within nurses' scope of practice

272

Documentation of Treatment Refusal

- Reasonable approaches of care refused:
  - ➤ Treatments
  - ➤ Procedures
  - ➤ Interventions

- Require prompt communication with care provider

273

Documentation of Errors

Should errors be documented?

How should they be documented?

A reasonable approach . . .

274

Areas of Liability and Patient Harm

- Telephone triage

- Obstetrical triage

- FHR interpretation, communication, and documentation

-Simpson, 2014

275

Areas of Liability and Patient Harm

- Elective induction of labor

- Cervical ripening

- Labor induction/augmentation

-Simpson, 2014

276

Areas of Liability and Patient Harm

- Tachysystole
- Pain relief during labor and birth
- Nurses role during regional anesthesia/ analgesia
- Fundal pressure in second stage labor

-Simpson, 2014

277

_____

_____

_____

_____

Areas of Liability and Patient Harm

- Shoulder dystocia
- Second stage labor management
- Forceps and vacuum assisted birth

-Simpson, 2014

278

_____

_____

_____

_____

Areas of Liability and Patient Harm

- Trial of labor after cesarean birth (TOLAC)
- Multiple gestation

-Simpson, 2014

279

Areas of Liability and Patient Harm

- Iatrogenic prematurity
- Perinatal GBS
- Neonatal resuscitation at birth
- Staffing

-Simpson, 2014

280

Leslie's Case

- 23 and 3/7 weeks gestation
- $G_1 P_0$
- Gestational hypertension
- Five prenatal visits:
  - O+; Rubella immune; RPR-NR, HbSAg-neg; HIV-negative
  - + Chlamydia; treated 2 months ago
  - Weight 140 pounds (8 lbs. gained during pregnancy)

281

Leslie's Case

- Family history:
  - Mother with chronic hypertension
  - Father with type II diabetes
  - Sister had preeclampsia 2 years ago
- Medical history:
  - Appendectomy at age 15 years
- Social history:
  - Unmarried, lives with her parents
  - Smokes ½ pack cigarettes daily; denies drug use

282

Leslie's Case

- Admitted to community hospital:
  - ➤ Elevated blood pressure at MD office
    - 162/100 after previous ranges of 109/65 to 126/64
  - ➤ Lab values:
    - CBC: WBC 13.9; Hgb 12.7; Hct 36.8
    - Platelets 206,000
    - CMP: normal
- Prior to transport received:
  - ➤ First dose betamethasone
  - ➤ Magnesium sulfate 4 g load/2 g hourly
  - ➤ Labetalol 20 mg IV push

283

Leslie's Case

- Blood pressures prior to transport
  - ➤ 152/86 to 159/92
- Vital signs during transport in same range
- Magnesium sulfate infusing at 2 g / hour
- Six or less contractions per hour

284

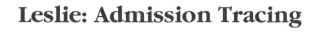

Leslie: Admission Tracing

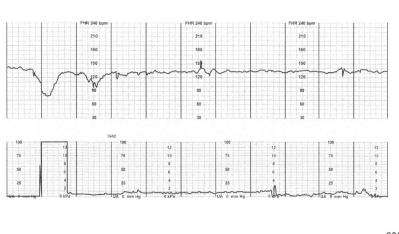

285

Leslie: Admission Tracing

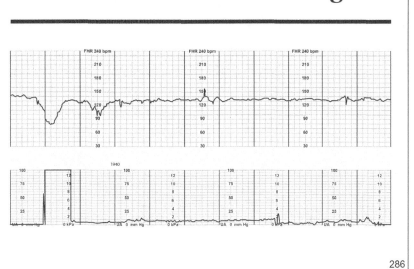

286

Leslie: 7 Minutes Later

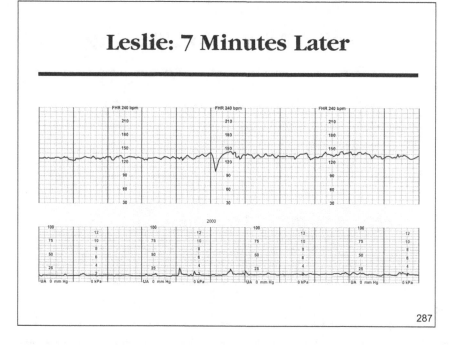

287

Tracing Prior to Monitor Removal

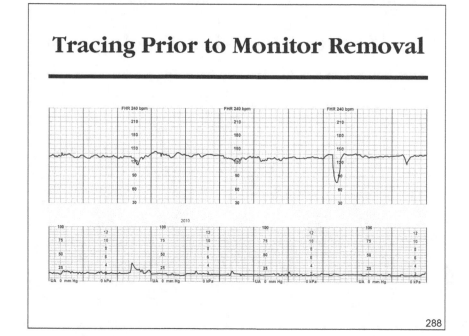

288

Leslie: Ultrasound Report

- Cephalic, gestational age 23.3 weeks
- Posterior placenta with multiple hypoechoic lesions measuring 2–3 cm
- Not typical for placental lakes
- EFW 1 lb. 4 oz. (35th percentile)
- Lagging abdominal circumference
- AFI 10.4 cm
- Fetus active

289

Tracing 3 Hours After Ultrasound

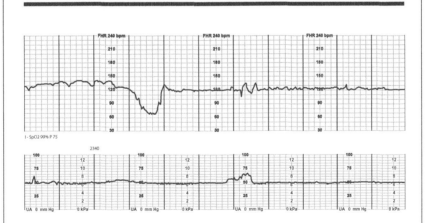

290

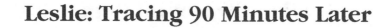

Leslie: Tracing 90 Minutes Later

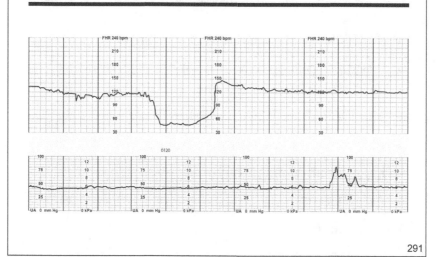

291

Leslie: Nine Hours After
Admission to Referral Hospital

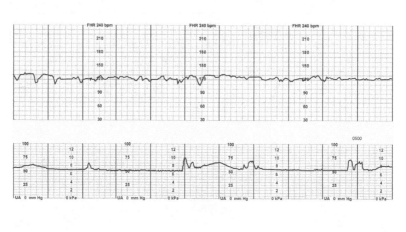

292

Perinatologist's Note

- Active problems:
  - ➤ IUP 24 w4d
  - ➤ Gestational hypertension
  - ➤ Placental disorder-suspect insufficiency
  - ➤ Hypoechoic lesions throughout placenta

- Has been normotensive since arrival

- Lab studies normal

293

Perinatologist's Note

- FHR pattern:
  - ➤ Intermittent decelerations:
    - ■ The latest two decelerations were 6 hours apart
    - ■ Tracing reactive for gestational age
    - ■ At times more reactive than at others
    - ■ Not frequent enough to warrant delivery
- Plan of care:
  - ➤ Administer second dose of steroid
  - ➤ Administer magnesium sulfate for neuroprotection
  - ➤ NPO

294

Nine Hours Later

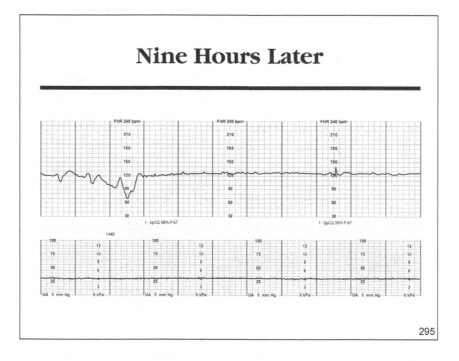

295

Leslie: Monitoring Continued

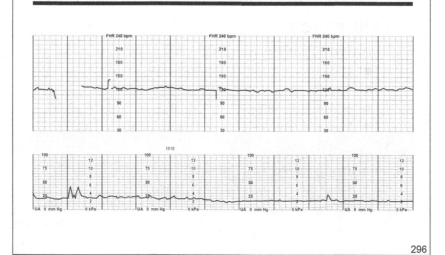

296

Leslie: Third Day at Referral Hospital

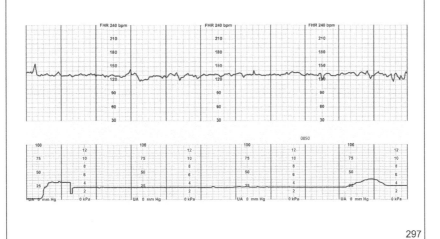

297

Leslie: Tracing 5 Minutes Later

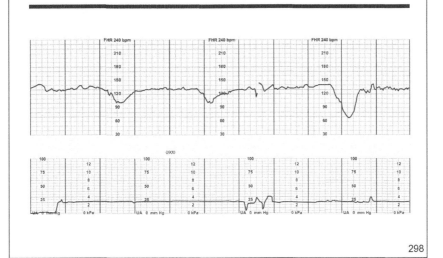

298

Ongoing Monitoring

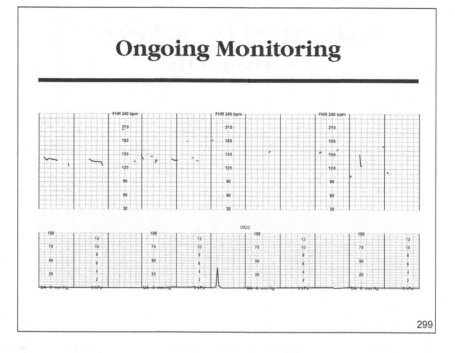

299

Leslie: Tracing, One Hour Later

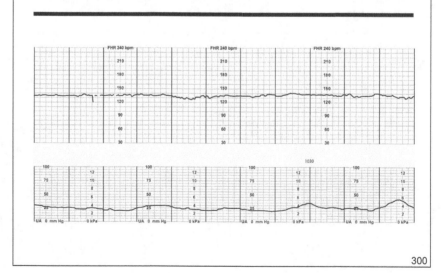

300

Leslie: Hospital Day Four

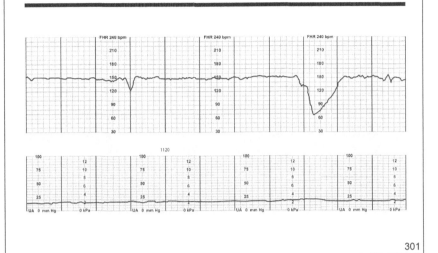

301

Prior to EFM Removal

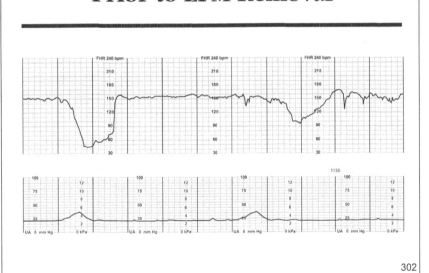

302

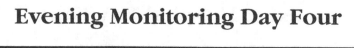

Evening Monitoring Day Four

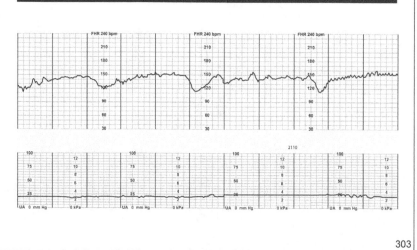

303

Day Four Evening Monitoring

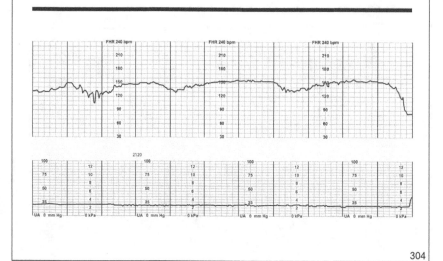

304

Forty Minutes Later

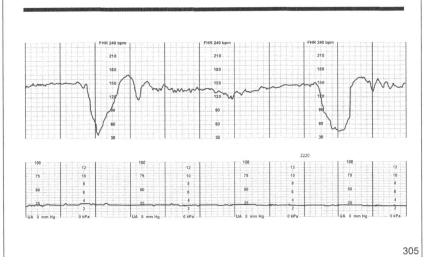

305

Leslie: Hospital Day Five

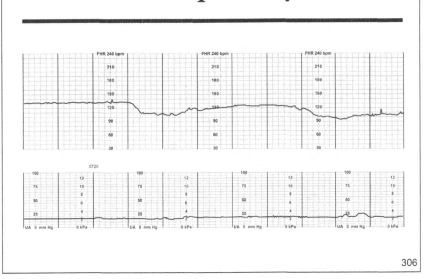

306

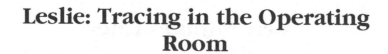

Leslie: Tracing in the Operating Room

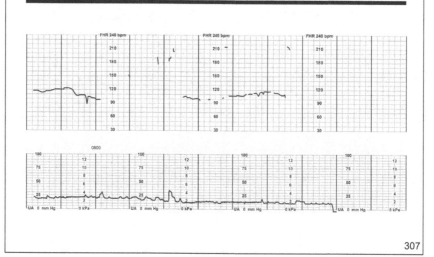

307

Leslie: Outcome

- Delivered male infant by cesarean @ 0810
- Apgar scores: 2/6/8 @ 1, 5, 10 minutes
- Weight: 1 lb. 1.6 oz.
- Umbilical arterial cord gas:
  ➤ pH 6.720
  ➤ Base excess –22
  ➤ CO_2 49
- Infant expired on day six of life secondary to severe intraventricular hemorrhage and extreme prematurity

308